Understanding
RESPIRATORY
MEDICINE

a problem-oriented approach

Edited by:

Martyn R Partridge
**Professor of Respiratory Medicine, Imperial College,
NHLI Division and Honorary Consultant Physician,
Charing Cross Hospital, London, UK**

With contributions by:

Dr Frances Bowen

Dr Robina Coker

Dr Andrew Cummin

Dr Philip Ind

Dr Claire Shovlin

Dr Mangalam Sridhar

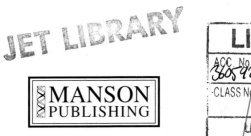

**MANSON
PUBLISHING**

Copyright © 2006 Manson Publishing Ltd

ISBN: 1-84076-045-1
ISBN 978-1-84076-045-3

A CIP catalogue record for this book is available from the British Library.

For full details of all Manson Publishing Ltd titles please write to:
Manson Publishing Ltd, 73 Corringham Road, London NW11 7DL, UK.
Tel: +44(0)20 8905 5150
Fax: +44(0)20 8201 9233
Website: www.mansonpublishing.com

Commissioning editor: Peter Altman
Project manager: Ruth Maxwell
Copy-editor: John Forder
Cover photograph and design: Cathy Martin, Presspack Computing Ltd
Book design and layout: Cathy Martin, Presspack Computing Ltd
Colour reproduction: Tenon & Polert Colour Scanning Ltd, Hong Kong
Printed by: Replika Press PVT Ltd, India

Contents

Preface

Respiratory diseases are common and affect large numbers of people. Care for those with respiratory illness is given by a multi-disciplinary team involving more than just doctors and nurses. This short textbook on respiratory medicine is intended as a practical guide to help those who care for adult patients with respiratory disease. It is aimed especially at senior medical undergraduates, junior doctors, and specialist nurses, but it is also intended for use by physiotherapists, physiological measurement technicians, and clinical scientists. Suggested sources for further reading are given where appropriate and websites from which you can download most of the major respiratory guidelines are listed below.

The book has been written by the senior staff of the NHLI Division of Imperial College, London working in the Department of Respiratory Medicine at the Charing Cross and Hammersmith Hospitals. I am grateful to my colleagues for meeting the deadlines associated with multi-authorship textbooks and to the publishers for their expert help.

Martyn R Partridge

Contributors

Dr E Frances Bowen (Chapters 4, 5, and 9), Consultant Physician and Honorary Senior Lecturer, Charing Cross and Hammersmith Hospitals

Dr Robina Coker (Chapters 3 and 8), Consultant Physician and Honorary Senior Lecturer, Hammersmith and Charing Cross Hospitals

Dr Andrew Cummin (Chapters 4 and 12), Consultant Physician and Honorary Senior Lecturer, Charing Cross Hospital

Dr Philip Ind (Chapters 7 and 15), Senior Lecturer and Honorary Consultant Physician, Hammersmith Hospital

Professor Martyn R Partridge (Chapters 1, 2, 7, and 11), Professor of Respiratory Medicine, Imperial College, NHLI Division and Honorary Consultant Physician, Charing Cross Hospital

Dr Claire Shovlin (Chapters 3, 14, and Glossary), Senior Lecturer and Honorary Consultant Physician, Hammersmith Hospital

Dr Mangalam Sridhar (Chapters 6, 10, and 13), Consultant Physician and Honorary Senior Lecturer, Charing Cross Hospital

Further sources of information

The British Thoracic Society website – www.brit-thoracic.org.uk – contains downloadable copies of British Thoracic Society guidelines on the following subjects:
   Asthma
   Chronic Obstructive Pulmonary Disease
   Pneumonia
   Pneumothorax
   Tuberculosis
   Diffuse Parenchymal Lung Disease
   Malignant Mesothelioma
   Pulmonary Embolus
   Fitness to Dive
   Fitness to Fly
   Non-Invasive Ventilation in Acute Respiratory
      Failure
   Pulmonary Rehabilitation
   Bronchoscopy
   Pleural Diseases

The Asthma UK website – www.asthma.org.uk – contains numerous patient information sheets, and also downloadable asthma self-management education materials.

The British Lung Foundation website – www.lunguk.org – contains patient information and information about nationwide 'Breathe Easy' clubs.
Other useful respiratory websites include:
   The Global Initiative for Asthma:
      www.ginasthma.com
   The Global Initiative for Obstructive Lung
      Disease: www.goldcopd.com
   The Lung and Asthma Information Agency:
      www.laia.ac.uk
   QUIT – the UK charity that helps people give up
      smoking: www.quit.org.uk
   Pneumotox website – www.pneumotox.com –
      collates reports of drug-induced lung disease.

Glossary

GENERAL SIGNS

Cachexia: This term describes weight loss and muscle wasting, usually due to an underlying malignancy. Muscle wasting may be recognized by its tendency to exaggerate the prominence of the skeleton.

Clubbing: Loss of the nailbed angle, and in later stages drumstick appearances, indicate clubbing (3.1). The earliest stage involves softening of the nailbed, which can be detected by rocking the nail from side to side on its bed. Clubbing is best seen by viewing the nail from the side against a pale background.

The mechanism by which clubbing develops is unknown. It occurs in the context of several serious respiratory conditions including lung cancer, chronic suppurative disease and right-to-left shunts. It may also reflect disease in other organs (particularly cardiac and gastrointestinal) and may be congenital, when it is entirely benign.

Horner's syndrome: This comprises miosis (contraction of the pupil), enophthalmos (backward displacement of the eyeball in the orbit), anhidrosis (lack of sweating on the affected side), and ptosis (drooping of the upper eyelid), usually due to involvement of the sympathetic chain on the posterior chest wall by a bronchial carcinoma.

Obesity: Obesity can be defined by reference to the body mass index (BMI), which is the weight (in kg) divided by the square of the height in metres. More sophisticated measurements of muscle and fat status (not performed as part of a routine respiratory examination) include triceps skinfold thickness and mid-muscle circumference. However, obesity carries significance in respiratory medicine because it is a cause of breathlessness, and because of its association with obstructive sleep apnoea (OSA). Excessive daytime drowsiness, night-time snoring, and early morning headaches are particularly suggestive of OSA or the obesity/hypoventilation syndrome.

Sputum: Sputum production is not normal. White (mucoid) sputum is produced in smokers, and in bronchitis. Thick, yellow or green (purulent) sputum usually indicates infection, but may be seen in asthma due to the presence of eosinophils. The yellow/green tinge reflects the presence of white blood cells. Blood-stained sputum varies from a rusty colour (in pneumonia) to frank blood, which must be investigated promptly as it is often due to lung cancer or tuberculosis.

IMPAIRED GAS EXCHANGE

Cyanosis: Reduced haemoglobin (mean capillary value of deoxygenated Hb ≥ 4 g/dl [or rarely methaemoglobin ≥ 0.5 g/dl]) gives a blue colour to the skin and mucous membranes. This approximates to an oxygen saturation of < 85%, but can occur at a higher saturation if the overall Hb is higher (in polycythaemic as opposed to anaemic patients). Only central cyanosis (when the oral mucous membranes appear blue) indicates respiratory disease and impaired gas exchange. Peripheral cyanosis, when the hands and feet are blue but the tongue is pink, is due to circulatory insufficiency.

Hypercapnoeic flap: This describes a flapping tremor of the outstretched hands (identical to that seen in hepatic failure). It is associated with carbon dioxide retention and may be seen in severe chronic obstructive airways disease. It is associated with warm peripheries indicating vasodilatation, a bounding pulse, papilloedema, and headache.

CHEST WALL ABNORMALITIES

Barrel chest: The chest wall is held in hyperinflation and the anteroposterior diameter of the chest is increased such that it may exceed the lateral diameter. The patient may well be using their accessory muscles of respiration.

Kyphosis: This is forward curvature of the spine. It may suggest osteoporotic vertebral collapse in a patient on long-term steroid therapy.

Pectus carinatum ('pigeon chest'): In pectus carinatum the sternum and costal cartilages project outwards. It may result from severe childhood asthma.

Pectus excavatum ('funnel chest'): The sternum is depressed in this condition, which is benign and requires no treatment. It can, however, distort chest radiographic appearances by making the heart appear enlarged and displaced to the left.

Scoliosis: This describes lateral curvature of the spine, which can lead to respiratory failure.

Tietze's syndrome: This term describes swelling of one or more of the upper costal cartilages in a patient with anterior chest pain, often exacerbated by unaccustomed exercise. In practice it is rare to find swelling and much more common to find tenderness on palpation unaccompanied by swelling.

PATTERNS OF RESPIRATION

Cheyne–Stokes respiration: This is a cyclical waxing and waning of the depth of breathing over 1–2 minutes, from deep respirations to almost no breathing. Two patterns are recognized: the first has a longer cycle (45 s to 2 minutes) and is due to a prolonged circulation time between the lungs and chemoreceptors: this usually reflects a circulatory problem, commonly due to left ventricular failure. The second pattern, of shorter cycles, is associated with respiratory failure due to impaired central control (including the effects of drug overdose). This pattern may also be observed during sleep.

Kussmaul respiration: This deep sighing pattern of respiration is seen in acidotic patients, typically from diabetic ketoacidosis but also in renal failure and after overdoses of aspirin. It may also be seen in patients with acute massive pulmonary embolism.

Respiratory rate: An increase in the rate and depth of breathing can occur in any severe lung disease and in fever. Prolonged hyperventilation (as seen, for example, in the course of a panic attack) causes a metabolic alkalosis secondary to lowering of the partial pressure of carbon dioxide in the blood. This, in turn, can result in acute hypocalcaemia, manifest as parasthesiae around the mouths, fingers, and toes, and positive Chvostek's and Trousseau's signs due to increased irritability of nerves and muscles.

To elicit Chvostek's sign, tap over the facial nerve in front of the ear. If positive, this will result in a brief twitch of the corner of the mouth on the same side. To elicit Trousseau's sign, inflate a sphygmomanometer cuff to just above systolic pressure for approximately 2 minutes. If positive, this will result in carpopedal spasm of the hand, with opposition of the thumb, extension of the interphalangeal joints, and flexion of the metacarpophalangeal joints. There is spontaneous resolution when the cuff is deflated.

PULMONARY CIRCULATION

Cor pulmonale: This is right-sided heart failure resulting from lung disease (see Chapter 6, page 53). The commonest cause in developed countries is chronic obstructive pulmonary disease. Signs of cor pulmonale include a raised jugular venous pulse, peripheral oedema, and a left parasternal heave, indicating right ventricular hypertrophy. If severe there may be functional tricuspid regurgitation causing a pulsatile liver, large 'v' waves in the jugular venous pulse and a systolic murmur in the tricuspid area.

RESPIRATORY MEASUREMENTS

Forced expiratory volume in 1 second (FEV_1): This is the volume of air expelled in the first second of a forced expiration, starting from full inspiration.

Vital capacity (VC): The total volume of air expelled in a forced expiration, starting from full inspiration.

FEV_1/VC ratio: The percentage of the VC exhaled in the first second of the forced expiration. In most normal subjects over 75% of the FVC would have been exhaled within 1 second.

Total lung capacity (TLC): This is the volume of gas in the lungs after a maximal inspiration (TLC = RV + VC).

Residual volume (RV): This is the volume of gas in the lungs at the end of a maximal expiration.

Abbreviations

(anti-)GBM = (anti-)glomerular basement membrane
(NF-kappa B) = nuclear factor-kappa B
AAFB = acid or alcohol fast bacillus
ABPA = allergic bronchopulmonary aspergillosis
ACA = anticentromere antibody
ACE = angiotensin converting enzyme
ADH = antidiuretic hormone
AFB = acid/alcohol-fast bacillus
AIA = aspirin-induced asthma
ALS = acute life support
ANA = antinuclear antibody
ANCA = antineutrophil cytoplasmic antibody
AP = anterior/posterior
AP-1 = activated protein-1
APTT = activated partial thromboplastin time
APUD = amine precursor uptake and decarboxylation
ARDS = acute respiratory distress syndrome
ASD = atrial septal defect
AV = alveolar volume
BAL = bronchoalveolar lavage
BCG = bacillus Calmette–Guérin
BHL = bilateral hilar lymphadenopathy
BMD = bone mineral density
BOOP = bronchiolitis obiliterans organizing pneumonia
BP = blood pressure
cAMP = cyclic adenosine monophosphate
CAP = community-acquired pneumonia
CCDC = Centres of Communicable Diseases Control
CFA = cryptogenic fibrosing alveolitis
CFC = chlorofluorocarbon
CNS = central nervous system
COAD = chronic obstructive airways disease
COLD = chronic obstructive lung disease
COP = cryptogenic organizing pneumonia
COPD = chronic obstructive pulmonary disease
COX(-1) = cyclo-oxygenase(-1)
CPAP = continuous positive airway pressure
CRP = C-reactive protein
CSF = cerebrospinal fluid
CSS = Churg–Strauss syndrome
CT = computed (axial) tomography
CT-PA = computed tomography pulmonary angiogram
CURB = confusion, urea, respiratory rate, blood pressure

CWP = coal worker's pneumoconiosis
DEXA = dual energy X-ray absorption (scan)
DOT = directly observed therapy
DPLD = diffuse parenchymal lung disease
DSCG = disodium cromoglycate
DVT = deep venous thrombosis
EAA = extrinsic allergic alveolitis
ECG = electrocardiogram
ECP = eosinophil cationic protein
EIA = exercise-induced asthma
EPX = eosinophil protein X
ESR = erythrocyte sedimentation rate
FBC = full blood count
FDG = fluorodeoxyglucose
FDG-PET = fluorodeoxyglucose positron emission tomography
FEV_1 = forced expiratory volume in 1 second
FRC = functional residual capacity
GR = glucocorticoid receptor
GRE = glucocorticoid response element
HFA = hydroxyfluororalkane
HHT = hereditary haemorrhagic telangiectasia
HMW = high molecular weight
HOA = hypertrophic osteoarthropathy
HPS = hepatopulmonary syndrome
HRCT = high-resolution computed tomography
ICS = inhaled corticosteroid
Ig(AEG) = immunoglobulin-(AEG)
INR = international normalized ratio
IPF = idiopathic pulmonary fibrosis
IVC = inferior vena cava
JVP = jugular venous pressure
KCO = transfer coefficient for carbon monoxide
LDCT = low-dose computed (axial) tomography
LDH = lactate dehydrogenase
LMW = low molecular weight
LT = leukotriene
LTOT = long-term oxygen therapy
LTRA = leukotriene receptor antagonist
LVF = left ventricular failure
LVRS = lung volume reduction surgery
MAI = *Mycobacterium avium-intracellulare*
MBP = major basic protein
MCP = monocyte chemotactic protein
MDR-TB = multi-drug resistant TB
MDT = multi-disciplinary team
MI = myocardial infarction
MRC = Medical Research Council

MRI = magnetic resonance imaging
MRSA = methicillin-resistant *Staphylococcus aureus*
NA = noradrenaline
NICE = National Institute for Clinical Excellence
NIPPV = noninvasive positive pressure ventilation
NOTT = Nocturnal Oxygen Therapy Trial
NP = nosocomial pneumonia
NRT = nicotine replacement therapy
NSAID = nonsteroidal anti-inflammatory drug
NSCLC = nonsmall-cell carcinoma (or nonsmall-cell lung cancer)
NSE = neurone specific enolase
OSA = obstructive sleep apnoea
PA = posteroanterior
pANCA = antineutrophil cytoplasmic antibody
PAS = para amino salicylic acid
PAVM = pulmonary arteriovenous malformation
PC = provocative concentration
PCR = polymerase chain reaction
PD = provocative dose
PDA = patent ductus arteriosus
PDE = phosphodiesterase
PE = pulmonary embolus
PEF = peak expiratory flow
PEFR = peak expiratory flow rate
PET = positron emission tomography
PG = Prostaglandin
PH = pulmonary hypertension
PKA = protein kinase A
pMDI = pressurized metered dose inhaler
PPD = purified protein derivative
PPH = primary pulmonary hypertension
PTH = parathyroid hormone
PTHrP = parathyroid hormone-like related peptide

PTR = partial thromboplastin ratio
PUO = pyrexia of unknown origin
RA = rheumatoid arthritis
RADS = reactive airways dysfunction syndrome
RANTES = regulated on activation normal T expressed and secreted
RAST = radioallergosorbent test
RBBB = right bundle branch block
RV = residual volume
SCA = squamous cell antigen
SCF = supraclavicular fossa(e)
SIADH = syndrome of inappropriate antidiuretic hormone secretion
SLE = systemic lupus erythematosus
SPN = solitary pulmonary nodule
SVC = superior vena cava
SVCO = superior vena cava obstruction
TB = tuberculosis
TGF-β = transforming growth factor-β
TH2 = T helper cell
TLC = total lung capacity
TLCO = transfer factor for the lung for carbon monoxide
TNAB = transthoracic needle aspiration biopsy
TNF = tumour necrosis factor
UIP = usual interstitial pneumonia
U&E = urine and electrolytes
VQ (scanning) = ventilation–perfusion (scanning)
VATS = video-assisted thoracoscopic surgery
VC = vital capacity
VSD = ventricular septal defect
WBC = white blood cells
WHO = World Health Organization
ZN = Ziehl–Neelsen (stain)

Chapter 1
AN OVERVIEW OF LUNG DISEASE

Chapter 2
THE SYMPTOMS OF LUNG DISEASE: TAKING THE RESPIRATORY HISTORY

Chapter 3
THE SIGNS OF LUNG DISEASE: THE RESPIRATORY EXAMINATION

Chapter 4
RESPIRATORY INVESTIGATIONS

LUNG FUNCTION TESTS

THORACIC IMAGING

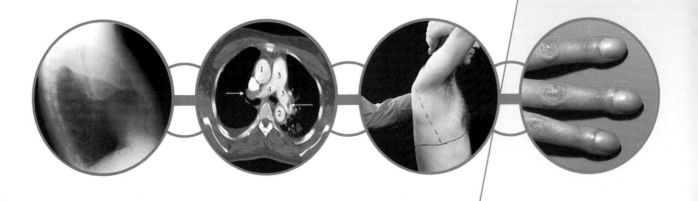

Chapter 1 An overview of lung disease

INTRODUCTION

The subject of respiratory medicine is bedevilled by indecision as to the name of the speciality. *Respiratory* physicians, known as *pulmonologists* in some countries, work in *chest* clinics where they utilise *lung* function tests and order *thoracic* computed tomography (CT) scans. In fact these terms are largely interchangeable, but it is important to state that this book on respiratory medicine is concerned with the diagnosis and management of adults with diseases that predominantly affect the lung, pleura, and chest wall.

THE SIZE OF THE PROBLEM

Respiratory diseases are large in number and affect sizeable numbers of the population. In the UK:

❑ Respiratory diseases account for one in four of all deaths.
❑ Lung cancer is the commonest cause of cancer death in both males and females.
❑ The most commonly reported long-term illnesses in children are conditions of the respiratory system.
❑ Respiratory disease is the most common illness responsible for an emergency admission to hospital.
❑ Respiratory disease is the most common reason to visit a general practitioner – more than a third of people will visit their general practitioner at least once a year because of a respiratory condition.
❑ While the death rate for heart disease has declined by 53% over the last 30 years, that for lung disease has stayed stubbornly steady. Indeed some diseases, such as asthma, have increased in prevalence over the last 30 years, and tuberculosis (TB) notifications have risen by 22% over the last 10 years, but this is not uniformly distributed geographically. Mesothelioma, a malignant tumour of the pleura, is causing a current epidemic of deaths reflecting exposure to asbestos 20–40 years ago, and it is estimated that this malignancy will continue to kill increasing numbers of people over the next two decades.

Deaths from lung disease in the UK tend to be higher than elsewhere in continental Europe, and while such comparisons clearly depend upon the accuracy of death certificates, the gap between the UK and countries such as Austria, Italy, Greece, and Germany is large and cannot be explained by smoking habits.

The morbidity associated with respiratory disease is also considerable and the World Health Organization (WHO) has predicted that chronic obstructive pulmonary disease (COPD), for example, will move from being the twelfth commonest cause of disability-adjusted life years lost in 1990, to being the fifth commonest cause (after ischaemic heart disease, depression, road traffic crashes, and cardiovascular disease) by 2020. 2,800,000 hospital bed-days are used every year in the UK for COPD and chest infections alone, and respiratory diseases cost the health service more than any other disease area.

Further data regarding the size of the problem of lung disease in the UK can be found by reading 'The Burden of Lung Disease', which may be accessed and downloaded from the British Thoracic Society's website (www.brit-thoracic.org.uk). Further UK data are available from the Lung and Asthma Information Agency (www.laia.ac.uk). Global data for the common diseases of asthma and COPD can be found on the websites of the Global Initiative for Asthma (www.ginasthma.com) and the Global Initiative for Chronic Obstructive Lung Disease (www.goldcopd.com). The WHO website (www.who.int/en/) is another useful source of data regarding the epidemiology and burden of lung diseases.

THE DIVERSITY OF RESPIRATORY CONDITIONS

There are more than 30–40 common respiratory illnesses, and it is important for the clinician to appreciate this, and not to think instantly of the commoner two or three to account for their patients' symptoms. Indeed, it is also important to remember that the symptoms of lung disease, such as breathlessness, are also shared with disorders of other systems (see Chapter 2, page 12) and may reflect lung disease, heart disease, pulmonary emboli, diaphragm weakness, or systemic disorders, such as anaemia or obesity. With such a large number of diseases it is important to have an overview of them all and to then take a structured approach to diagnosis. An overview of all respiratory conditions is shown in *Table 1*.

DIFFERENTIATION BETWEEN OBSTRUCTIVE AND RESTRICTIVE (SMALL-LUNG) DISORDERS AND ACCURATE DIAGNOSIS

Once infectious diseases and pulmonary emboli have been excluded, the traditional classification of lung diseases is into restrictive and obstructive lung disorders. The word restrictive does not carry any particular meaning to most clinicians, and it is therefore better to think of this group of disorders as being small-lung disorders. However, as *Table 1* emphasizes, such small lungs may reflect disease of the lungs themselves, or processes going on around the lungs, such as pleural disease, chest wall deformity or diaphragm weakness. Obesity as a cause of breathlessness is often overlooked in this context and is a potent cause of both small lungs and impaired function, as well as imposing additional respiratory workload.

Differentiation into obstructive disorders and small-lung disorders may be made in the traditional way by means of history and clinical examination; or the process may be obvious on a chest radiograph, which may clearly show small lungs in a case of obesity, and large lungs with hyperinflation in someone with severe airway obstruction and gas trapping. However the ultimate arbiter is the use of spirometry and other tests of lung function, and obstructive and restrictive (small-lung) spirometric results are discussed in Chapter 4, page 26.

LIVING WITH LUNG DISEASE

While some respiratory illnesses, such as pneumonia, post-viral cough, or pulmonary emboli may be isolated incidences occurring only once in a person's lifetime, many are long-term conditions which the patient has to learn to live with. Some, such as asthma, have the potential to be well controlled, albeit with regular medication, but others, such as COPD and diffuse parenchymal lung disease, may be associated with persistent disability. Some of these diseases particularly affect those also suffering socio-economic deprivation. Some which are associated with smoking are associated with depression and stigma and the realization that the condition is self-induced. Others, such as lung cancer, cystic fibrosis, and mesothelioma are associated with significant reduction in life expectancy.

For all these reasons it is essential that those caring for those with lung disease understand the need for good communication, the need to demonstrate empathy and support, and the need for what is often called 'holistic care'. Such care is increasingly given in a multi-disciplinary manner and the team is likely to involve primary care physicians, practice nurses, chest physicians, specialist respiratory nurses, physiotherapists, pharmacists, clinical scientists, Macmillan nurses, and physiological measurement technicians.

Table 1 An overview of respiratory diseases

Infections
- ❏ Infective bronchitis
- ❏ Pneumonia
- ❏ Empyema
- ❏ Tuberculosis

Airway diseases
- ❏ Localized
  - Obstructive sleep apnoea
  - Laryngeal carcinoma
  - Thyroid enlargement
  - Vocal cord dysfunction
  - Relapsing polychondritis
  - Bronchial carcinoma
  - Tracheal carcinoma
  - Carcinoid tumour
  - Adenoid cystic carcinoma
  - Post tracheostomy stenosis
  - Foreign bodies
  - Bronchopulmonary dysplasia
- ❏ Generalized
  - Asthma (including occupational asthma)
  - COPD
  - Bronchiectasis
  - Cystic fibrosis
  - Obliterative bronchiolitis

Small-lung disorders
- ❏ Lung diseases
  - Sarcoidosis
  - Asbestosis
  - Extrinsic allergic alveolitis (e.g. bird-fancier's lung, farmer's lung, mushroom packer's-lung)
  - Fibrosing alveolitis
  - Eosinophilic pneumonia
- ❏ Pleural diseases
  - Effusions
  - Pneumothorax
  - Mesothelioma
- ❏ Chest wall/muscle disease
  - Scoliosis
  - Respiratory muscle weakness
- ❏ Other
  - Obesity

Pulmonary vascular disorders

Chapter 2 The symptoms of lung disease: taking the respiratory history

INTRODUCTION

A history is taken from patients in order to make a diagnosis. Indeed, history taking should permit us to construct a reasonably accurate diagnosis or differential diagnosis in over 90% of cases. Clinical examination may subsequently confirm either normality or the suspected diagnosis, but only occasionally elicits anything unexpected. If, at the end of history taking, a differential diagnosis has not been formulated, clinical examination alone is unlikely to shed light upon the pathological problem and further history taking followed by investigation is necessary.

A respiratory history should include details of symptoms suggestive of respiratory pathology, a general history, and also specific reference to the smoking history, occupational history, environmental history, and family history.

SYMPTOMS OF RESPIRATORY DISEASE

BREATHLESSNESS

Breathlessness, or dyspnoea, is a sensation of difficult, laboured or uncomfortable breathing. Sometimes it is referred to as 'air hunger'.

Breathlessness may reflect:
- Physiological causes:
  – Strenuous exercise.
  – Pregnancy.
- Psychological causes:
  – Stress.
  – Anxiety.
  – Panic attack.
- Pathological causes: with regard to pathological causes, it is very important to remember that breathlessness may be due to:
  – Lung disease.
  – Heart disease.
  – Pulmonary vascular disease.
  – Neuromuscular disease (e.g. diaphragm weakness).
  – Systemic disorders (for example, anaemia, hyperthyroidism, obesity).

When assessing the breathless patient one should enquire about:
- The onset of breathlessness (e.g. acute, gradual)?
- The circumstances of the breathlessness (e.g. on exertion or at rest)?
- Worse at night?
- Worse on lying flat?
- Associated symptoms?
- Severity of breathlessness?

Careful determination of the onset of breathlessness and its timing and circumstance may be crucial with regard to the causation of that symptom. *Box 1* contains a checklist of possible causes of breathlessness, the onset of which may be within a few moments, over hours or days, or over weeks, months or years. When using this list, it is important to remember that patients sometimes adapt their lives to cope with a symptom, and may believe it to be of more recent onset than is the real case. It is sometimes worth seeking clarification by asking questions such as 'Can I just check that this time last year you could have run upstairs as quickly as me?' or 'Can I just check that last month you were able to do all your usual activities including making the bed, carrying the shopping?' It is also important to be able to grade the severity of the breathlessness, and while several such grades are available, one of the most commonly used is the Medical Research Council's dyspnoea grade, which is shown in *Table 2*.

Further necessary questions regarding the symptom of breathlessness relate to factors which make the

---

BOX 1 The differential diagnosis of breathlessness according to the onset of that symptom

Within minutes: Pulmonary embolus, pneumothorax, myocardial infarction (MI), cardiac rhythm disturbance, dissecting aneurysm, acute asthma.

Over hours or days: Pneumonia, pleural effusion, left ventricular failure (LVF) (LV dysfunction, valve dysfunction or septal rupture post MI), asthma, blood loss, lobar collapse, respiratory muscle weakness (Guillain–Barré syndrome).

Over weeks: Infiltration (malignancy, sarcoidosis, fibrosing alveolitis, extrinsic allergic alveolitis, eosinophilic pneumonia), respiratory muscle weakness (motor neurone disease), main airway obstruction, anaemia, valvular dysfunction.

Over months: Same as for weeks plus obesity, muscular dystrophy, asbestos-related conditions.

Over years: Chronic obstructive pulmonary disease (COPD), chest wall deformity, heart valve dysfunction, obesity.

> **Table 2 Medical Research Council dyspnoea grade**
> 1 Normal
> 2 Able to walk and keep up with people of similar age on the level, but not on hills or stairs
> 3 Able to walk for 1.5 km on the level at own pace, but unable to keep up with people of similar age
> 4 Able to walk 100 m on the level
> 5 Breathless at rest or on minimal effort

symptom worse, and it is important to determine whether this symptom is present only on exertion, or whether it is present at rest. For example, patients with COPD are only usually breathless at rest when they have very advanced disease, and in most cases have their worst symptoms on exertion, even simple exertion such as dressing. By contrast, the person with asthma may be well for most of the time but during an exacerbation they may have severe breathlessness even at rest; characteristically the breathlessness wakes them during the night and is present – and often at its worst – on waking in the morning.

All diseases capable of causing breathlessness can be made worse by the recumbent posture, a reflection of the mechanical disadvantage at which accessory muscles work on lying down and of the pressure of the abdominal contents upon the diaphragm. Marked worsening on lying flat is often referred to as orthopnoea, and this symptom is often regarded as being pathognomic of heart failure. While this is very often the cause of this symptom, it should also be remembered that rarely orthopnoea may be a presenting feature of diaphragm failure, such as that which may occur with post-infectious ascending polyneuritis (the Guillain–Barré syndrome), or with the amyotrophic lateral sclerosis form of motor neurone disease.

COUGH

A cough is a powerful reflex response designed to protect the lungs from the noxious effects of inhaled foreign substances, both mechanical and chemical. It is a rapid, intensely forceful movement and the cough airflow may exceed 12 l/sec. A cough, like the symptom of breathlessness, may be quantified and one such quantification is shown in *Table 3*.

The commonest cause of an acute short-lived cough is an acute viral infection, but a cough may reflect the presence of a number of airway diseases and small-lung disorders. A cough may therefore be a feature of:

❏ Laryngeal carcinoma.
❏ Tracheal carcinoma.
❏ Bronchial carcinoma.
❏ Bronchial carcinoid.
❏ Asthma.
❏ COPD.
❏ Bronchiectasis.
❏ Cystic fibrosis.
❏ Foreign body inhalation.

However, a cough is also a prominent feature of infection, such as:

❏ Infective bronchitis.
❏ Tuberculosis.
❏ Pneumonia.

A cough is also a distressing feature of many small-lung disorders, especially:

❏ Fibrosing alveolitis.
❏ Sarcoidosis.
❏ Extrinsic allergic alveolitis.
❏ Eosinophilic pneumonia.
❏ Asbestosis.

Always be concerned by a patient, especially a smoker or an ex-smoker, who presents with a new onset cough or a change in character of a long-standing cough. Such patients need a chest radiograph to exclude lung cancer.

It is also important to remember that 10–20% of patients started on an angiotensin converting enzyme (ACE) inhibitor may develop a cough, and the temporal association between the introduction of these drugs and the onset of the symptom is not always close.

Table 3 A scheme for the quantification of cough

Score	Daytime	Night-time
0	No cough	No cough
1	Cough for one short period	Cough on waking only, or on going to sleep only
2	Cough for more than two short periods	Woken once, or woken early owing to cough
3	Frequent cough not interfering with usual activities	Frequent waking due to coughing
4	Frequent cough interfering with usual activities	Frequent cough most of the night
5	Distressing cough most of the day	Distressing cough

A chronic cough is usually defined as a cough lasting for 2 months or more. If the chest radiograph is normal, five common causes are:

❑ Smoking.
❑ Eosinophilic bronchitis.
❑ Post-nasal drip (from associated rhinosinusitis).
❑ Asthma.
❑ Gastro-oesophageal reflux.

With regard to the latter, it is important to remember that a cough may reflect gastro-oesophageal reflux without the patient necessarily complaining of any associated heartburn.

Cough with sputum production

Small amounts of phlegm may be produced in many conditions including:

❑ Smoking.
❑ COPD.
❑ Infective bronchitis.
❑ Lung cancer.
❑ Asthma.

Production of large amounts of phlegm may reflect an origin in the upper airways and reflect the presence of sinus disease. However, if more than a teaspoonful of sputum is produced every day and there is no evidence of sinus disease, then it is important to consider the possibility of bronchiectasis, cystic fibrosis or other suppurative lung diseases (see Chapter 11, page 119).

HAEMOPTYSIS

Haemoptysis, or the coughing up of blood, should always be taken seriously and regarded as reflecting significant pathology until proved otherwise. Occasionally it is difficult to be certain of the origin of blood which appears in the mouth, and if the blood is fresh and unaltered by contact, for example, with acid, then an origin in either the upper gastrointestinal tract,

an oral origin, or a lung origin are all possible. Blood mixed with sputum is perhaps the commonest presentation and this signifies an airway origin, which may be in the upper or lower airways. There are many possible causes, but as a minimum this symptom necessitates careful history taking to determine other significant features, careful examination, and a chest radiograph. Depending upon the clinical circumstance, and frequency of the symptom, further invasive and radiological investigations may also be indicated. Possible causes of haemoptysis are listed in *Table 4*.

CHEST DISCOMFORT

The character, site, radiation, aggravating and relieving features of any chest discomfort should be determined, as should duration and the presence or otherwise of associated symptoms.

Minor chest discomforts are not uncommon and often reflect a musculoskeletal origin, sometimes associated with physical exertion and sometimes associated with violent coughing. Occasionally violent coughing can lead to rib fractures and these are usually associated with intense pain on coughing and movement or pressure upon the chest, over the site of the fracture. Occasionally, direct extension of tumours into the chest wall may be associated with continuous, pressing pain, and occasionally metastases occur to the rib from primary tumours, both within and without the chest. The most specific respiratory cause of chest discomfort is that of pleuritic pain, which reflects friction between the visceral and parietal pleura as they move over one other during respiration. Pleuritic pain is usually sharp, stabbing, and worse on inspiration, and it is important to remember that it may reflect infection or infarction. The common causes of pleuritic pain are thus:

❑ Pneumonia.
❑ Pulmonary embolus and infarction.
❑ Pneumothorax.
❑ Malignancy.

Table 4 Possible causes of haemoptysis

❑ Bronchial carcinoma/tumours	❑ Goodpasture's syndrome
❑ Tuberculosis	❑ Pulmonary endometriosis
❑ Bronchiectasis	❑ Coagulopathies
❑ Cystic fibrosis	❑ Mitral valve disease
❑ Lung abscess	❑ Left ventricular failure
❑ Pulmonary infarction	❑ Iatrogenic causes
❑ Pneumonia	❑ Biopsy
❑ Mycetoma	❑ Drugs (anticoagulants, aspirin)
❑ Pulmonary arteriovenous malformations	

Pleurisy may also occur in other inflammatory conditions, such as rheumatoid arthritis and systemic lupus erythematosis.

WHEEZING, MUSICAL BREATHING, STRIDOR, AND HOARSENESS

The term wheeze is probably medical jargon, and while it is entering the lay vocabulary, it is not often offered as a spontaneous symptom. While often associated with asthma, patients with asthma more often complain of coughing, chest tightness, and breathlessness, but may describe musical breathing or a high-pitched noise coming from the chest (wheezing). This is usually most marked on breathing out. Wheezing reflects vibration of an inflamed airway wall and does not necessarily equate with airway narrowing, nor indeed with any one specific pathology. Simple viral infections may lead to wheezing, and wheezing can be a prominent symptom in COPD as well as in asthma; its presence does not imply the likelihood of reversibility of airway narrowing. Similarly severe airway narrowing can be present without the presence of wheezing.

Stridor has a lower pitch than wheezing and is maximal on inspiration. It is usually a finding on examination, rather than a spontaneously offered symptom, but occasionally patients are aware of and complain of a harsh noise on inspiration. Stridor indicates a likely obstruction of the main airway or larynx, and is usually heard best without the stethoscope.

Hoarseness may reflect either pathology of the larynx or damage to its nerve supply. Lung pathology may account for the latter; the long course of the left recurrent laryngeal nerve, which comes down into the chest and passes round the left hilar structures, is often subject to pressure from bronchial carcinomas either directly from the tumour itself, or by compression by secondary malignant lymphadenopathy. All hoarseness needs to be taken seriously and investigated but one of the key features of the hoarseness associated with recurrent laryngeal nerve palsy is that it is a loss of volume to the voice as much as a change in character of the voice. Patients often complain most of not being able to make themselves heard on the telephone or above ambient noise, and they also have an ineffectual cough because they are unable to close their cords to build up sufficient intrathoracic pressure.

SNORING AND EXCESSIVE DAYTIME SLEEPINESS

40% of the population snore, but 5% of an adult population may also have obstructive sleep apnoea syndrome (see Chapter 12, page 124). This condition is associated with repetitive obstruction of the upper airway during sleep; patients suffer repeated arousal and do not achieve deep sleep, with the result that they experience excessive sleepiness the next day. It is important to be able to quantify the degree of sleepiness suffered by such patients, and to distinguish clearly between the symptom of sleepiness and that of a feeling of tiredness. Sleepiness may be quantified by use of the Epworth sleepiness scale, which is shown in *Table 5*.

Table 5 The Epworth sleepiness scale

In contrast to just feeling tired, how likely are you to doze off or fall asleep in the following situations? Even if you have not done some of these things recently, try to work out how they would affect you. Use the following scale to choose the most appropriate number for each situation: 0 = no chance of dozing; 1 = slight chance; 2 = moderate chance; 3 = definitely would doze.

Situation	Chance of dozing	Situation	Chance of dozing
Sitting and reading:		Lying down to rest in the afternoon when circumstances permit:	
Watching TV:		Sitting and talking to someone:	
Sitting inactive in a public place (e.g. theatre or a meeting):			
		Sitting quietly after lunch without alcohol:	
As a passenger in a car for an hour without a break:		In a car while stopped for a few minutes in traffic:	

OTHER FEATURES OF THE RESPIRATORY HISTORY

SMOKING HISTORY

Smoking accounts for well over 90% of all cases of bronchial carcinoma, and well over 90% of COPD. It also significantly increases the risk of carcinoma of the nasal passages, mouth, tongue, and larynx and is a potent risk factor, for example, for postoperative chest infections. While it is very important to take a full smoking history in every patient, it is obviously especially important to explore this subject in those with probable respiratory disease. This can best be undertaken by remembering the '5 As' in *Box 2*.

PASSIVE SMOKING (BREATHING SECOND-HAND SMOKE)

It is also very important to ask about passive smoking. While transient exposure to environmental tobacco smoke, for example in a public house, may be an irritant and may provoke symptoms in somebody with asthma, a more significant risk arises in those who are living or working over long-term periods with smokers. There is now compelling evidence that passive smoking is a cause of lung cancer and studies comparing nonsmoking women who live with smokers compared to those who live with nonsmokers have shown an excess risk of lung cancer of up to 24%. This corresponds to hundreds of deaths due to lung cancer in the UK every year as a consequence of breathing other peoples' smoke. It has also been suggested that the risk of ischaemic heart disease amongst nonsmokers living with smokers, compared to those who live with nonsmokers, may be 25% higher – which equates to half the risk of smoking 20 cigarettes a day.

SMOKING CESSATION

Most smokers wish to give up smoking. The vast majority say they would not smoke if they had their time again, and the biggest reason for this is concern regarding health. While continued smoking is more common in those who suffer socio-economic deprivation, the motivation to quit is identical in all social classes. All health care professionals need to give clear, unequivocal, nonjudgmental advice to smokers about the need to stop. If patients express a willingness to stop smoking, they need to be given specific advice as to how to do so, how to cope with withdrawal symptoms, how to access nicotine replacement therapies and other medications, and all need to be reminded of the benefits of stopping.

OTHER ENVIRONMENTAL HISTORY

In addition to a properly taken smoking history, a more detailed environmental history is also necessary in patients with several respiratory diseases. It is very important for those with asthma to identify factors in their environment which may have precipitated worsening of their symptoms, and this may include anything from exposure to pets to cleaning out dusty areas, to use of aspirin or nonsteroidal anti-inflammatory agents or to sleeping on a bottom bunk and being showered with house dust mite when the older sibling turns over during the night. It is also important to enquire about hobbies. For example, delays in the diagnosis of extrinsic allergic alveolitis may occur if a history of the keeping of pigeons, cockatiels or other birds is not elicited.

BOX 2 Checklist for the evaluation of smoking history – the '5As'

1 Ask
- ❏ Establish smoking history – smoker, nonsmoker, or ex-smoker?
- ❏ Record status in notes.

2 Advise
- ❏ Explain the value of stopping and the risks to health of continuing.
- ❏ Personalized – taking account of:
  – Existing conditions or family history.
  – Early signs of disease.
  – Impact on others, including children.
  – Financial consequences.

3 Assess – establish an interest in stopping:
- ❏ 'How do you feel about your smoking?'
- ❏ 'Have you ever tried to stop?'
- ❏ 'Are you interested in stopping now?'

4 Assist – help should be offered to those who want to quit:
- ❏ Set a date and plan for it.
- ❏ Avoid smoking situations (e.g. pubs).
- ❏ Involve partner, friends, family.
- ❏ Review past experience – what went wrong?
- ❏ Refer on for more counselling – specialist service?
- ❏ Prescribe nicotine replacement therapies or buproprion.

5 Arrange follow-up

OCCUPATIONAL HISTORY

Occupational lung diseases are becoming more common and are often associated with a delay in diagnosis. Occupational lung diseases include:

- ❏ Occupational asthma.
- ❏ Lung cancer secondary to asbestos, cadmium, chromium, and nickel exposure.
- ❏ Asbestos-related lung disease.
- ❏ Other pneumoconioses and dust-related diseases.
- ❏ Pigeon-fancier's lung.
- ❏ Granulomatous lung disease, e.g. berylliosis.
- ❏ Farmer's lung.

Occupational causes may account for 3–5% of all cases of asthma and, indeed, in any adult presenting with asthma who does not have any early life history of the condition, one should always be suspicious of an occupational or environmental cause. Some common causes are shown in *Table 6* but it should be stressed that new agents capable of causing occupational asthma are being identified all the time and the possibility of an occupational cause for the disease should always be borne in mind. It can be helpful specifically to ask the patient if they have noted whether they are better at weekends or when away on holiday, and if there is any suspicion of occupational asthma the patient should be referred to an expert in occupational lung disease.

ASBESTOS-RELATED LUNG DISEASE

During the first decade of the 21st century, there is an epidemic of deaths related to asbestos exposure 20–40 years ago. Occupations involving exposure to asbestos include:

- ❏ Asbestos industry (mining, manufacture).
- ❏ Naval dockyard workers.
- ❏ Dock workers in general.
- ❏ Builders, laggers, plumbers, demolition workers, electricians, and boilerhouse men.
- ❏ Brake lining manufacturers.
- ❏ *And the wives and families of the same who may have been exposed to asbestos brought home on working clothes.*

Expose to asbestos may lead to:

- ❏ Pulmonary fibrosis (asbestosis).
- ❏ Benign pleural plaques.
- ❏ Pleural malignancy (mesothelioma).
- ❏ Diffuse pleural thickening.

These diseases are considered further in Chapters 8 and 9.

Additional tips on taking a history are given in *Box 3*.

Table 6 Common causes of occupational asthma (and occupation/activity associated with it)

- ❏ **Chemicals,** such as colophony (soldering), isocynates (car paint spraying), and drugs (penicillin) in occupations such as, for example, dye workers, foam manufacture
- ❏ **Grains and plants,** e.g. wheat (millers), flour (bakers)
- ❏ **Insects,** e.g. locusts (lab workers)
- ❏ **Animals,** e.g. rats, mice (lab workers), avian proteins (bird fanciers)
- ❏ **Fungi,** e.g. mushroom spores
- ❏ **Metals,** e.g. platinum (refiners), cobalt (grinders), stainless steel (welders)
- ❏ **Enzymes,** e.g. *Bacillus subtilis* (detergent manufacturers)

BOX 3 Tips on taking histories and presenting findings

Although the history is recorded in the order described in the previous section, the order in which the information is obtained may be different. For example:

- ❏ Patient rapport may be helped if one starts with the friendly aspects of the social history.
- ❏ Much of the information obtained later in the history may be relevant to the *history of the presenting complaint.*

It may be useful to finish with a question like *'Is there anything else we haven't covered?'* in case the patient's memory has been jogged or more trust has been gained.

For this reason it is often worth reorganizing the history after the details have been taken from the patient. This is often best done *before* the patient is examined so that the clinician has an idea of what signs to look for.

Abbreviations should not be used in case records – what is written should be understandable by all who read the records, including the patient.

Chapter 3 The signs of lung disease: the respiratory examination

INTRODUCTION

THE FIVE GROUPS OF SIGNS
- General: cachexia/obesity; tar-stained fingers; clubbing; sputum; lymphadenopathy.
- Signs of impaired gas exchange: central cyanosis; hypercapnoeic flap.
- Chest wall abnormalities and pattern of respiration: chest wall abnormalities may be primary, or secondary to, underlying lung disease; respiratory rhythm and rate.
- Focal respiratory signs: abnormal percussion, vocal resonance and auscultation due to abnormalities of the airways, parenchyma, or pleural disease. This is the most extensive section and most feared by students!
- Right heart signs: raised jugular venous pressure; peripheral oedema; right ventricular heave; palpable or loud pulmonary second sound.

METHOD OF EXAMINATION

GENERAL APPROACH
1 After your history review, or when meeting a patient for first time, ask their permission to examine them and ask them to undress to the waist. Ask female patients to remove their bra and provide them with a blanket. A chaperone may be required – ask the patient. You may need nursing assistance if the patient is in a wheelchair or finds undressing difficult (you should note if they are breathless while undressing).
2 Sit the patient at 45° in a comfortable position on the examination couch.
3 Next proceed to a careful general inspection from the end of the bed:
   - First look round to see if inhaler, nebulizer, sputum pot or oxygen mask are present.
   - Then look at the patient, noting their general appearance (e.g. cachexia, central cyanosis, breathlessness).
   - Count the respiratory rate over 15 seconds (without the patient being aware that you are counting).
4 Examine the hands, noting the presence or absence of the following:
   - Tar staining from cigarettes.
   - Finger clubbing (1).
   - Tremor (may indicate treatment with β_2 agonists).
   - Hypercapnoeic flap: ask the patient to hold out their arms and extend their wrists, keeping their fingers apart, and observe for a flapping tremor. Assess over at least 5 seconds.
   - Blueness of fingers (indicating peripheral cyanosis).
   - Thin skin and bruising (may indicate long-term steroid therapy).
5 Begin your detailed examination of the chest. This should follow the standard pattern of inspection, palpation, percussion, and auscultation.

Inspection
Remember surface anatomy considerations (2). From the end of the bed, first ask the patient to take a single deep breath. As they do so, note the presence or absence of the following:
- Symmetry of chest wall movement on deep breathing (the side which moves less has the pathology).
- Chest wall deformities (pigeon, funnel, etc.).
- Barrel chest, hyperinflation, or use of accessory muscles of respiration.
- Scars (may indicate previous surgery or invasive procedures such as chest drain insertion).
- Enlarged veins over the chest (should raise suspicion of superior vena caval obstruction).
- Symmetry and any skin changes over the breasts (men as well as women).

Palpation
Measure chest expansion
This is done by placing your hands symmetrically on each side of the chest and comparing the degree of

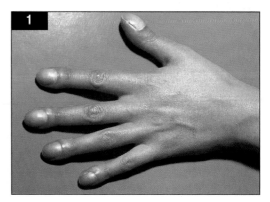

1 Finger clubbing

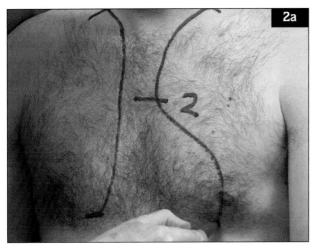

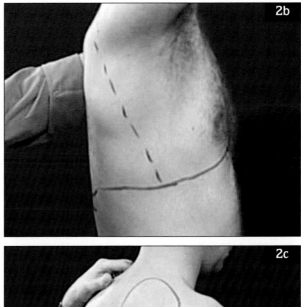

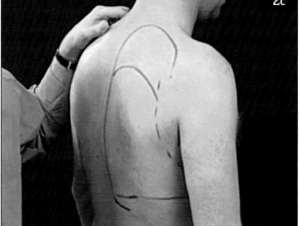

movement on each side when the patient takes a deep inspiration (3). It is best to ask the patient to 'breathe in, breathe out [position hands on chest now] and breathe in again'. To position your hands, place your fingers horizontally facing posteriorly and pull your thumbs forward to the anterior midline; they should be nearly touching in the anterior midline following the deep expiration. Subtle changes can be detected, especially if the hands are initially placed as posteriorly as possible. Repeat anteriorly and posteriorly over the lower zones of the chest. For the upper zones you may find that placing your hands vertically is more helpful, but best of all is a good look. Reduced movement on one side suggests pathology on that side and is extremely helpful in interpreting subsequent signs.

2 Surface anatomy of the chest. (**a**), Anterior: the sternal angle indicates the position of the second rib. The lung extends to the eighth rib laterally and tenth rib posteriorly. (**b**), Position of the oblique fissure. (**c**), Position of the right upper and lower lobes

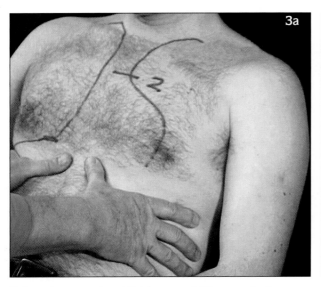

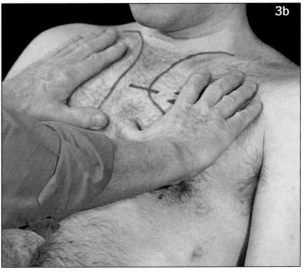

3 Assessing expansion of (**a**) lower and (**b**) upper chest

Determine the position of the apex beat

The apex beat may be shifted towards the side of collapse or fibrosis of either lower lobe, or away from the side of a pleural effusion or pneumothorax.

Examine the ribs and the sternum for swelling and tenderness

Marked tenderness, sometimes with swelling of the costo-chondral joints of the upper ribs, and occasionally also the sterno-clavicular joints, may arise in Tietze's syndrome. Swelling and tenderness of the ribs and sternum are also common in metastases, myeloma, and leukaemia.

Determine the position of the trachea

This is one of the most important clinical signs in chest disease, and may, for example, be the only clue to fibrosis of an upper lobe. The patient should be sitting up with the neck slightly flexed and not rotated. We think that the easiest method is to insert the index and middle fingers in the suprasternal notch and feel for tracheal displacement. Warn the patient that this may feel a little uncomfortable.

Examine for enlarged cervical lymph nodes

Stand just in front of, and later behind, the sitting patient. Use a slow and gentle sliding or rotary motion of the palmar aspect of the finger tips, not heavy pressure. Remember that the sternomastoids divide the neck into anterior and posterior triangles, and be methodical.

Have a definite and fixed order for palpation of the individual groups of nodes: occipital, post- and pre-auricular, submandibular, submental, anterior triangle and posterior triangle, and supraclavicular. If enlarged nodes are found, note their size, consistency, and whether fluctuant, tender, mobile, discrete or matted, and whether they are attached to the skin or other structures. If any enlarged cervical nodes are found, the area of their lymphatic drainage should be explored and a search made for other enlarged nodes in the axillae, epitrochlear, and inguinal regions.

Examine for enlarged axillary lymph nodes

The method is similar to that for the cervical nodes. Face the seated patient and support the patient's arm; start high in the axilla and bring your fingers slowly down while exerting a constant gentle pressure against the chest wall.

Examine the breasts

You are not usually expected to examine the breasts as part of a supervised respiratory examination, but the method is included here for the sake of completeness. You should become familiar with the technique, and with normal and abnormal findings. It may yield vital information in the assessment of a respiratory patient, such as the presence of an unexplained pleural effusion.

The breasts should be palpated with the palmar aspect of the middle three fingers, using one hand only. Move your hand in a circular movement while exerting at first gentle and later increasingly firm pressure against the chest wall. Examination of each quadrant must be carried out in turn. If the breasts are pendulous, it may be better for the patient to lean forward slightly. It often helps if the breasts are examined with the patient's hands clasped behind her neck. Stand on the patient's right side to examine the right breast and on her left for her left breast. Any breast swelling that can be felt with the flat of the hand is likely to be neoplastic. Gynaecomastia may be seen in men with intrathoracic malignancy.

Assess vocal fremitus

Vocal fremitus assesses the transmission of low-frequency voice sounds through the lung. They are transmitted better by consolidated lung, but poorly by pleural effusions. The transmission of sounds is felt by your hand when the patient loudly and deeply repeats a phrase such as '99'. You must compare the corresponding parts of the right and left sides of the chest using the same hand, as your hands may not be equally sensitive. If you are not sure of your findings the first time, don't despair. Vocal resonance is easier to assess (see below) and repetition of attempts at vocal fremitus are unlikely to be helpful. You should attempt this a maximum of three times anteriorly and posteriorly.

Percussion

It is better to percuss with the patient sitting up rather than lying down (4). If the patient is too ill to sit up, percussion posteriorly should be done with the patient rolled onto each side in turn. It is important not to keep on tapping one area many times, because each tap will produce a different note and more uncertainty. Try to develop your technique so that you can give an opinion after, at most, two taps. Always compare the corresponding part of the chest on the opposite side, always with your finger in the intercostal space and equidistant from the midline.

One finger should be applied very firmly, either entirely in an interspace, or entirely along the rib percussed, but never across a rib. Use the pad of your finger on the other hand, not the tip, to make the percussion stroke. Make the stroke from the wrist and strike at right angles to the finger on the chest, using a short, sharp, and decisive stroke. Practise this first on a table and then on yourself – you will find that louder notes are obtained by increasing the pressure of the lower finger on the surface, rather than hitting it with increasing force with the upper finger. Keep your fingernails short.

The normal percussion note varies over different parts of the chest, being most resonant at the lung apices. You will need a good deal of practice to learn what constitutes a normal note at any area. Always move from resonant to dull, and compare right and left sides at each level. The percussion note may be increased or decreased. A hyper-resonant note is lower in pitch and more vibrant. Dullness indicates pathology, but resonance does not imply the absence of pathology.

Auscultation

First show the patient exactly how you wish him or her to breathe, deeply but not noisily, with the mouth open to minimize any sounds produced in the nose, but not attempting to force expiration. Place your stethoscope directly on the skin, choosing the least hairy areas as far as possible (5). Warm your stethoscope diaphragm first if it is cold.

Characterize the breath sounds
Breath sounds are generated by turbulent flow in large airways. Detection at the surface implies that these have passed through the intervening lung tissue. Normal lungs filter out high frequency sounds: during a normal breath, the inspiratory sound is followed immediately without an interval by a shorter expiratory sound. Some have likened it to the noise made by wind rustling in the trees.

Bronchial breathing occurs because solid lung is better at transmitting high-frequency sounds. Bronchial breathing has a blowing quality, is louder, and higher pitched. Expiration is prolonged, and there is a short gap between inspiration and expiration. Higher-pitched vocal sounds are also better transmitted: whispering pectoriloquy refers to the ability to detect a whispered '22' with the stethoscope. To imitate bronchial breathing, place your tongue against the roof of the mouth and quietly blow in and out through your open mouth. Or you can whisper the word 'who'. Bronchial breathing is heard over consolidation but may also be found over collapse, at the top of an effusion or, rarely, over a cavity.

Determine the presence and nature of any added sounds
Wheezing is a high-pitched musical sound reflecting vibration in the walls of narrowed airways. It can sometimes be heard without a stethoscope in patients with bronchospasm, especially during a severe attack of asthma. Wheezes are monophonic when they have a single source and hence pitch, but more often they are polyphonic as they originate in many different-sized airways.

Crackles (crepitations) are interrupted 'popping' sounds heard mainly at the height of inspiration and the beginning of expiration, and are accentuated by coughing. They cannot be heard without a stethoscope. You can imitate them by rubbing

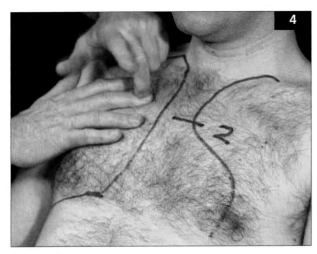

4 Percussion

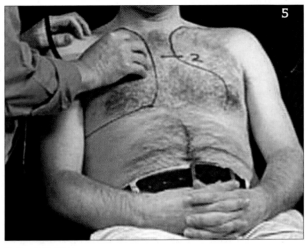

5 Auscultation

together the hairs near your ear. Crackles are most commonly associated with fluid in the airways and alveoli, and indicate a lung lesion which may be of any nature. Late inspiratory crackles indicate alveoli cracking open (for example, due to fibrosis) or fluid in the alveoli (resulting from pulmonary oedema).

Rhonchi are continuous sounds that diminish on coughing and are audible during most of inspiration and expiration. They are produced in the bronchi and indicate partial bronchial obstruction, usually due to upper airways secretions, the commonest cause of which is bronchitis.

A pleural rub is a squeaking sound rather like that produced by new leather. It is usually localized to a fairly small area and does not disappear on coughing.

Assess vocal resonance
Vocal resonance is the same as vocal fremitus (assessing the transmission of low-frequency voice sounds) but is elicited on auscultation rather than on palpation. It is performed by rapid comparison of the equivalent part of the chest on each side, while the patient says a deep and loud '99'. Consolidation is usually but not always associated with increased vocal resonance. In all other lung pathologies the usual finding is reduced vocal resonance in proportion to the degree of impairment of the percussion note.

Concluding steps
❑ Check for peripheral oedema and assess the jugular venous pressure (JVP).
❑ Check temperature, peak flow and sputum pot.
❑ Either at the beginning or at the end of your examination you should record the patient's weight.
❑ Consider whether your findings fit any recognized pathological pattern (6), and ask to recheck if in doubt.

6

	Normal	Consolidation	Pleural Effusion	Pneumothorax
Inspection				
Movement	Symmetrical			↓
Palpation				
Movements	Symmetrical	⇓	⇓	⇓
Tactile vocal fremitus	Symmetrical	↑	↓	↓
Percussion note	Symmetrical (resonant)	Dull	Stony dull	Hyper-resonant*
Auscultation				
Normal breath sounds	Normal	Bronchial	Bronchial or absent	↓
Added sounds	Nil	?Rhonchi	Nil	Nil
Vocal resonance		↑	↓	↓
Other		Pyrexia, sputum		

6 Overview of examination findings in common pathologies, best recognized when unilateral pathology results in asymmetrical signs. *Clue: the side that moves more sounds duller

CASE STUDIES

CASE STUDY 1

A 47-year-old shop assistant complains of chest pain and breathlessness. She last felt well 3 months ago. She is not sure whether it is the left-sided pain that increases when she coughs that has made her unable to walk round the shopping centre without stopping. Colleagues say she looks thin and poorly.

Question: What must you ask?

She admits to smoking 1–2 packs of cigarettes daily, managing to drop three dress sizes without dieting, and coughing up a little blood two days earlier.

Question: What must you look for on examination?

She is clubbed, cachectic, has tar-stained fingers, and an enlarged cervical lymph node. There are focal respiratory signs: the right lung displays reduced movement and a dull percussion note, and no breath sounds are audible.

Question: What is the likely diagnosis?

Lung cancer and malignant pleural effusion.

CASE STUDY 2

A 58-year-old man complains of cough, breathlessness, and ankle swelling. He admits that he always has a smoker's cough and needs antibiotics from his GP four or five times a year, but his cough is not much worse than usual. Over the last 2 weeks he has felt particularly short of breath and has been too chesty to walk to the pub. His wife is worried that his ankles look puffy for the first time.

Question: What are you particularly looking for on examination?

On examination he is coughing mucopurulent sputum, is cyanosed, and has tar-stained fingers. The chest is hyperexpanded with poor lateral expansion bilaterally. Widespread wheezes and crackles are audible. The JVP is elevated and peripheral oedema is present.

Question: What is the likely diagnosis?

Infective exacerbation of COPD and cor pulmonale.

CASE STUDY 3

A 68-year-old retired postman presents with a history of dry cough and increasing breathlessness over the last 18 months. He denies fever or weight loss but admits to intermittent joint pains in his hands. In the past his wife kept an aviary of budgerigars.

Question: What are you particularly looking for on examination?

Examination reveals a well-nourished man, not breathless at rest or on undressing, with finger clubbing and bilateral fine basal crackles.

Question: What is your differential diagnosis?

☐ *Cryptogenic fibrosing alveolitis.*
☐ *Rheumatoid arthritis with pulmonary fibrosis.*
☐ *Chronic extrinsic allergic alveolitis ('bird fancier's lung').*

ACKNOWLEDGEMENTS

2–5 are taken from the video 'Examination of the respiratory system', Medical Illustration Group 2001, Imperial College London, Charing Cross Hospital, editors Anthony Seed, Claire Shovlin, and Douglas Corfield.

Chapter 4 Respiratory investigations: lung function tests

INTRODUCTION

A wide variety of investigations test some aspect of lung function. Watching a patient walk or climb stairs is a test of cardiopulmonary function and quite a good one. A patient who can run up a flight of stairs is unlikely to have much functional impairment of either the heart or lungs. Simple exercise studies have been formalized in tests, such as the 6-minute walk and shuttle tests, which enable the degree of functional impairment to be measured. The 6-minute walk is most suitable for patients whose exercise tolerance is very limited. The distance the patient can walk in 6 minutes provides a measure of the ability to exercise.

Shuttle tests can be used for a wide range of subjects, including the very fit, but have been adapted to make them more suitable for clinical work. The patient walks back and forth between two markers 10 metres apart in response to a pre-set timer. The timer beeps to indicate when the patient should have reached the marker. Gradually the beeps get faster and faster until the patient cannot keep up (7). The stage when they have to stop provides a measure of their ability to exercise. More sophisticated exercise tests are not usually necessary and are beyond the scope of this chapter, which focuses on the basic tests of lung function.

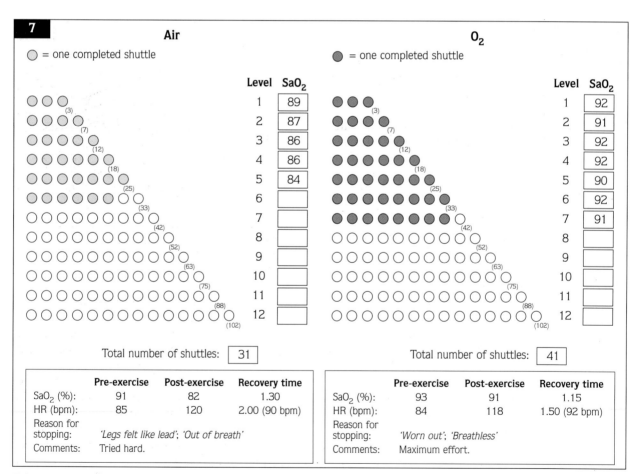

7 Shuttle exercise tests performed on a patient with severe emphysema. The first test was performed with the patient breathing air and the second test when breathing oxygen. Notice the improvement in the level of exercise she achieves when breathing oxygen, and the improvement in the oxygen saturation (SaO_2). HR, heart rate

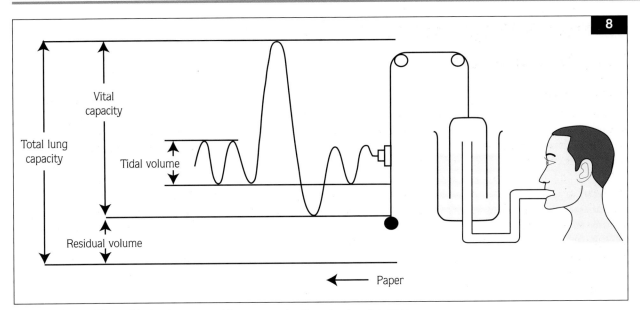

8 Lung volumes. The residual volume cannot be measured with a simple spirometer

NOMENCLATURE

The lungs are a reciprocal pump and their volume varies (**8**). When we breathe quietly a volume of air enters and leaves the lungs in a reasonably regular fashion. This is the tidal volume. When we exercise this volume will increase.

If we take in as large a breath as possible the lungs are then completely full. This volume, the volume of all the gas within the lungs, is known as the total lung capacity (TLC). If we then breathe out as far as we can some, but not all, of the air in the lungs is expelled. The volume we can breathe out is known as the vital capacity (VC). The volume left in the lungs at the end of a maximal expiration is the residual volume (RV).

VENTILATORY FUNCTION

Some lung volumes are very easy to measure. To measure the VC is simply a matter of measuring the volume of air that is breathed out following maximal inspiration. The instrument for doing this is known as a spirometer (**9**). There are various ways in which the volumes can be measured. In the wedge spirometer, the air blown into the tube fills a wedge bellows. As the wedge fills, a pen moves across graph paper on the top of the machine to indicate the volume.

Much more information can be obtained following a forced expiratory manoeuvre. The subject takes a deep breath in and then breathes out into the spirometer as fast and for as long as he can. The graph paper can be made to move as the patient

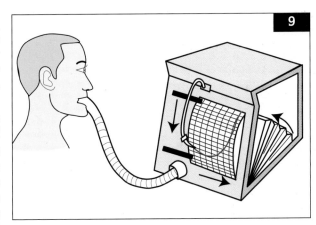

9 A normal subject using a wedge spirometer. At the beginning of the forced expiration the graph paper moves, enabling the FEV_1 to be measured

breathes out to produce a graph of volume against time. A normal subject can breathe out his whole VC within 3 seconds, and about three-quarters of this (75%) will be in the first second. To breathe out quickly the airways must be fully open. The flow of air out of the lungs is fastest at the beginning of forced expiration when the lungs and the airways within them are expanded, and slows to a stop at the end of expiration as the lungs and airways shrink. A patient with narrowed airways will not be able to breathe out so rapidly and the forced expiratory manoeuvre will take much longer. The volume breathed out in the first second is known as the forced expiratory volume in one second or, more usually, the FEV_1.

Unsurprisingly, this figure is reduced in patients with airway obstruction.

The FEV_1 is a very useful test for airway obstruction. But there is a problem. A patient with abnormally small lungs but no airway obstruction may also have a low FEV_1. How can we distinguish a patient with small lungs (a restrictive defect) from a patient with airway disease? For this we also need to take account of the VC. A patient with small lungs will have a small VC but, like a normal subject, will be able to breathe out most of this within the first second. On the other hand a patient with airway obstruction is unable to breathe out quickly and, unlike a normal subject or a patient with small lungs, will not be able to breathe out three-quarters of his VC in 1 second. For this reason it is helpful to express the FEV_1 as a percentage of the VC. If this is above 75% there is no airway obstruction. In this way spirometry, a simple, quick and cheap test, can distinguish between the two main types of defect: obstructive (resulting from narrowed airways) and restrictive (resulting from small lungs).

The output from a spirometer can be displayed in various ways. One standard method is to plot the volume the subject breathes out against time (**10**). In patients with an obstructive defect and a restrictive defect the VC is reduced. While it is important to look at the trace, not least to ensure that it is technically satisfactory, it is helpful to be able to record the results numerically. The key figures are the FEV_1, the VC, and the ratio FEV_1/VC. Examples from four patients are shown.

It is easy to understand why a patient with small lungs may have a reduced VC but what about the patient with airway obstruction? Patients with obstruction tend to have large lungs but they may be unable to empty them because of narrowed airways or loss of lung elasticity. In these patients there is gas trapping and the RV will be high.

It follows that a patient with a small VC may have either small lungs or airway obstruction. These two possibilities can be distinguished by looking at the FEV_1/VC ratio, but it would be ideal to know the size of the residual volume. The problem is that the RV cannot be measured with simple spirometry, though standard lung function laboratories are able to do this using dilution techniques or plethysmography.

Traditional spirometers display the results of the forced expiratory manoeuvre as a plot of volume against time (**10**), but modern electronics make it equally easy to plot flow against volume. This is usually combined with a forced inspiratory manoeuvre to produce what is known as a flow-volume loop.

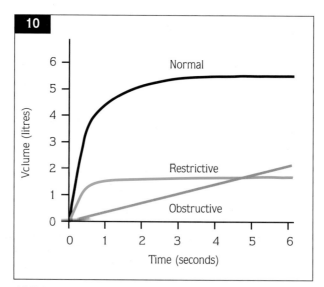

10 Spirometer traces from a normal subject, a patient with an obstructive defect, and a patient with a restrictive defect (small lungs)

CASE STUDIES

CASE STUDY 1

A 44-year-old man was sent for spirometry after complaining of breathlessness.

	Result	Predicted
FEV$_1$	4.9 l	3.9 l
VC	6.0 l	5.0 l
FEV$_1$/VC	82%	78%

Interpretation: These results are normal. There is no evidence of obstruction or small lungs (restriction). However, it is impossible to say that the patient has not got asthma, only that there is no evidence of asthma at the time of the test.

CASE STUDY 2

A 59-year-old man was complaining of breathlessness. The request form read '?asthma'.

	Result	Post-salbutamol	Predicted
FEV$_1$	1.6 l	2.3 l	2.9 l
VC	2.7 l	2.8 l	3.7 l
FEV$_1$/VC	59%	82%	78%

Interpretation: The initial spirometry showed obstruction, so the laboratory staff asked the patient to take some inhaled salbutamol and repeated the test after 10–15 minutes. The result was now normal. The airway obstruction was reversible, so this patient has asthma. If the patient had used his inhaler before the tests this diagnosis could not have been made.

CASE STUDY 3

A 75-year-old lady was sent to the laboratory from the cardiology department complaining of breathlessness on exertion. The request form read 'central cyanosis, clubbed, late inspiratory crackles, normal echocardiogram'.

	Result	Predicted
FEV$_1$	1.1 l	1.7 l
VC	1.2 l	2.4 l
FEV$_1$/VC	92%	71%

Interpretation: This patient's FEV$_1$ and VC are reduced but there is no evidence of obstruction. The FEV$_1$/VC is unusually high for a woman of this age. This suggests a restrictive (small lung) defect. The patient proved to have the cryptogenic fibrosing alveolitis form of diffuse parenchymal lung disease (see Chapter 8, page 81), which had been mistaken for heart failure.

CASE STUDY 4

A 51-year-old man was sent to the lung function laboratory with a request form which read simply '?emphysema ?pigeon fancier's lung'.

	Result	Predicted
FEV$_1$	1.8 l	3.5 l
VC	4.2 l	4.4 l
FEV$_1$/VC	43%	80%

Interpretation: The FEV$_1$ is reduced but the VC is normal. The FEV$_1$/VC is low. This is a picture of airflow obstruction which would be consistent with emphysema but not pigeon fancier's lung, which causes small lungs (restrictive defect). It is not possible to say more than this. The patient might have asthma and it would be important to go on to see if the airflow obstruction was reversible by testing the response to a bronchodilator.

An example of a normal flow-volume loop is shown by the solid loop in figure **11**. The subject takes a big breath in to TLC and then breathes out as fast and for as long as possible. When the lungs are fully expanded the airways are at their widest, so flow is at a maximum at the beginning of expiration. As the lung volume falls the airways become narrower and the flow falls progressively until flow ceases at RV. During inspiration the shape of the loop is different because the negative pressure within the thorax tends to open the airways, so that at the beginning of inspiration flow in is greater than the equivalent flow out.

If a patient has a rigid concentric tumour in the trachea, this will limit the maximum flow and the flow-volume loop will follow the dashed line. If a similar obstruction is less rigid it may be possible to determine from the flow-volume loop whether the obstruction is intrathoracic or extrathoracic. An intrathoracic obstruction will tend to be worse during expiration, when pressure within the thorax tends to worsen the narrowing, and better during inspiration, when the negative pressure tends to open the airway. The opposite will occur if the obstruction is extrathoracic.

More commonly the shape of the flow-volume loop may suggest loss of pulmonary elasticity and emphysema (**12**). Here, in the absence of normal elastic forces in the lungs to hold the airways open, the positive intrathoracic pressure associated with forced expiration causes the airways to collapse early in expiration, and from then on flow is severely reduced – 'pressure-dependent airway collapse'. The shape of the inspiratory loop is much more normal as the negative pressure tends to splint the airways open. Less severe airflow obstruction is characterized by a less severe 'scalloping' of the expiratory part of the loop – 'volume-dependent airway collapse'.

PEAK FLOW

During forced expiration the peak expiratory flow can easily be measured with a peak flow meter (**13**). These instruments are small, robust, and cheap but their application is limited. While it is self-evident that narrowing of the airways will lower the peak flow, patients who are unable to expand their lungs to a normal size may also have a low peak flow because small lungs have small airways. It follows that a single reading from a peak flow meter may not distinguish between the two main types of problem: airway obstruction and small lungs.

The simplicity and cheapness of the peak flow meter make it practicable for patients to perform the test at home over a period of time. Several readings

over time are much more valuable than a single test in the laboratory or GP's surgery. Indeed, some experts have suggested that spirometry should be the test

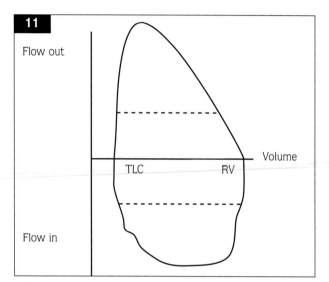

11 A normal flow-volume loop. The patient is asked to breathe in as far as possible, and then breathe out as fast and as far as he/she can. When expiration is finished, the patient takes a full breath in as fast as possible. The flow out is maximal when the airways are largest, and becomes progressively smaller as the lungs decrease in size. The inspiratory loop has a different shape. A rigid concentric tumour in the trachea would limit the flow as shown by the dotted line, and the flow-volume loop would take on a distinctive shape with expiratory and inspiratory plateaus. RV, residual volume; TLC, total lung capacity

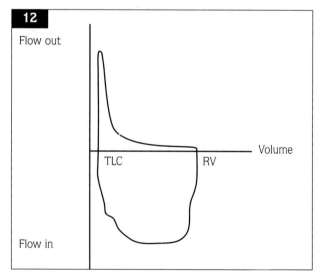

12 The shape of the flow-volume loop often seen in emphysema. As well as the shape of the curve being abnormal the actual flows are markedly reduced. The total lung capacity (TLC) and residual volume (RV) are increased

performed by the doctor in the clinic, hospital or the consulting room, and peak flow should be the measurement made by the patient in the home. Used in this way the simple peak flow meter can be used to diagnose asthma by detecting variability in airflow obstruction either spontaneously or in response to treatment – the key feature that characterizes asthma (see Chapter 7, page 60). The peak flow meter can also be used to monitor the severity of asthma and personalized asthma action plans can be based upon these readings (see Chapter 7, page 66). Used in this way, the peak flow meter is an excellent way of serially monitoring someone with known airway obstruction, but its value in diagnosis is limited.

LUNG VOLUMES

Using a simple spirometer it is easy to measure the VC. But after a full expiration there is still air left in the lungs and it would be helpful if we could measure this. In practice the volume measured is usually the functional residual capacity (FRC) from which the other lung volumes can easily be derived. At first sight this might appear to be difficult but a number of methods are available. One commonly used technique is helium dilution (**14**). If a patient's lungs are connected to a spirometer of known volume containing a known concentration of helium, the helium will become diluted by an amount dependent on the volume in the lungs. Helium is essentially insoluble in blood so measuring the final concentration of helium enables the lung volume at the time of connection to be calculated.

Measuring lung volumes is a useful adjunct to spirometry. For example it can be used to confirm small lungs (a restrictive defect). In airflow obstruction the VC may not give much of an indication as to the size of the lungs because the patient cannot breathe out as fully as normal. Some of these patients, for example those with emphysema, will have a large total lung capacity and their inability to breathe out as far as normal will be reflected in a high RV.

GAS TRANSFER

The gas transfer properties of the lungs can be tested by measuring the uptake of carbon monoxide, which is handled by the lungs in a similar manner to oxygen. In the UK a single breath method is commonly used. The patient breathes out fully then takes in a maximal breath of a gas mixture containing known concentrations of carbon monoxide (0.28%) and helium (14%) and holds his/her breath for 10 seconds to allow the carbon monoxide to diffuse into the pulmonary capillaries and the helium to mix within the lungs. As the patient breathes out the dead space is discarded, the alveolar gas is sampled, and the concentrations of carbon monoxide

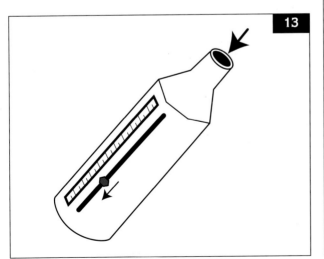

13 A peak flow meter. Useful to diagnose and monitor asthma

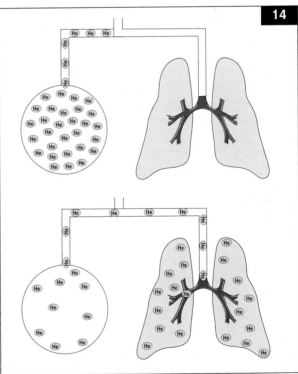

14 Lung volumes can be estimated using helium dilution. Helium is insoluble and will not be absorbed from the lung. The lung volume can be calculated from the fall in concentration of helium

and helium are measured. From the dilution of the helium the initial concentration of carbon monoxide entering the lungs can be calculated as can the alveolar volume (AV) (provided that the gas has been quickly and evenly distributed). The final concentration of carbon monoxide can be measured and, from this, the transfer factor for the lungs for carbon monoxide (TLCO) can be derived. This is a measure of how well the lungs as a whole take up carbon monoxide. The transfer coefficient (KCO) is a measure of how well each unit of lung to which the test gas has been distributed takes up carbon monoxide, and is obtained by dividing the transfer factor by the estimate of the AV.

A number of conditions interfere with this process. For example, impaired gas transfer may be seen in patients with fibrotic lung disease or emphysema or in anaemia (because there is less haemoglobin to take up the carbon monoxide). Pulmonary haemorrhage may cause increased carbon monoxide uptake. In conditions which prevent the lung from expanding, for example neuromuscular disease, the transfer coefficient may be very high because there is more blood flowing through a given volume of normal lung.

NORMAL RANGES

People vary in size and shape. Even when corrected for height, weight, and race, there is a considerable variation in lung volume from one individual to another. As a result the normal range for many lung function tests is wide. An exception, because it is a ratio, is the FEV_1/VC. As a rough rule the FEV_1 should not be less than 75% of the VC, but this too has a normal range, which falls with age. A peak flow that deviates slightly from the mean predicted may not be clinically significant. On the other hand a peak flow which falls significantly below an individual's personal known best is abnormal even if still within the normal range. It follows that, in a patient with known asthma, it is much more useful to ask the patient what their best ever peak flow is than to look up the normal value in tables.

PULSE OXIMETRY

Central cyanosis is an important clinical sign of arterial hypoxaemia but can be difficult to detect, especially in poor light. Small falls in saturation may not be detectable clinically but may be very important. A major advance has been the wide availability of pulse oximetry to measure arterial haemoglobin oxygen saturation.

The pulse oximeter is the ultimate safety monitor, as without either a pulse or oxygenation it will set off an alarm. This feature has probably saved countless lives. There is now such reliance on these instruments

that it is important to understand their operation and their limitations. Oximeters determine the haemoglobin saturation from the difference between the absorption spectra of oxygenated and deoxygenated haemoglobin. Modern pulse oximeters rely on just two wavelengths of light and are able to separate the pulsatile arterial signal from that of venous blood or tissues. The key components can be fitted into a small clip that will fit comfortably on the finger or ear.

It is important to interpret the results of oximetry in the context of basic physiology. For example, because of the shape of the haemoglobin dissociation curve, a small fall from normal saturation of 96% to 91% would reflect a large fall in arterial PO_2. This is of great clinical significance, not because a 5% fall in saturation matters to most patients, but because of the underlying cause. The response to such a fall in saturation would commonly be to give the patient oxygen. But it is important to consider the reasons for the desaturation. For example, giving oxygen to a patient with respiratory depression would bring about a rapid improvement in the oximeter reading but the patient would still be at risk if the underlying cause was not recognized. In a patient with COPD it might even exacerbate the problem.

Pulse oximeters are not always accurate. For example, they should never be used in suspected carbon monoxide poisoning because carboxyhaemoglobin is detected as oxygenated haemoglobin. The same phenomenon may cause over-reading in cigarette smokers.

ARTERIAL BLOOD GASES

The partial pressures of carbon dioxide and oxygen and the pH of arterial blood can readily be measured using a blood gas machine. A sample of blood is drawn, usually from the radial artery, into a heparinized syringe. It is essential to record the concentration of oxygen the patient is breathing. Any gas in the sample is expelled and the sample is transferred quickly to the analyser. Here the sample is brought into contact with electrodes sensitive to pH, PCO_2, and PO_2. From the measured variables the bicarbonate can be derived. Most blood gas machines also calculate the base excess. This is the difference between the derived bicarbonate and the bicarbonate that the computer calculates the patient should have assuming a normal metabolic acid–base state. The normal range for the base excess is -2 to +2 mmol/l. Anything outside this reflects a metabolic acid–base disturbance.

Blood gases are not quite as difficult to interpret as might appear from examples in some books; the clinical context usually gives some clues.

CASE STUDIES

CASE STUDY 5

This young woman was brought into the accident and emergency department semiconscious, having been found in her bedroom with an empty bottle of whisky and an empty bottle of sleeping pills alongside her. Arterial blood gases on air were:

	Result	Normal range
pH	7.16	7.38–7.42
PCO_2	10.7 kPa	4.8–5.9
PO_2	5.3 kPa	10.6–13.3
Base excess	+1.0 mmol/l	-2 to +2

Interpretation: The pH shows that the patient is acidotic. Is this the result of respiratory depression or has the patient taken, say, aspirin and developed a metabolic acidosis? The grossly raised PCO_2 shows that there must be at least an element of respiratory acidosis. But it is still possible that there is also an element of metabolic acidosis or that there may have been some metabolic compensation (though this seems unlikely as the clinical picture suggests an acute problem). The normal base excess shows that there is no metabolic acid–base disturbance and that this is an acute respiratory acidosis.

CASE STUDY 6

During cold weather a 74-year-old man was found semiconscious at home. Because he was known to attend the COPD clinic he was not given oxygen, and the following arterial blood gases were obtained:

	Result	Normal range
pH	7.36	7.38–7.42
PCO_2	8.0 kPa	4.8–5.9
PO_2	5.3 kPa	10.6–13.3
Base excess	+7 mmol/l	-2 to +2

Interpretation: Like patient 5 this patient is acidotic, though the pH is only slightly low. The nearly normal pH seems inconsistent with the PCO_2, which is high. The reason is found in the base excess, which shows that there has been some metabolic compensation. This implies that the respiratory acidosis is long-standing and is consistent with the apparent background of COPD. An interesting coincidence is that the PO_2 of this elderly man, who probably has COPD, is exactly the same as that of patient 5, a young woman, who probably has normal lungs. The reason is found in the PCO_2 values. The young woman has severe respiratory depression and this is the main cause of her hypoxia. The old man has a similar problem but it is less severe and his abnormal lungs are contributing to his hypoxaemia. This then is a compensated respiratory acidosis. Hypoventilation alone cannot account for the low PO_2.

CASE STUDY 7

A 34-year-old man arrived in the accident and emergency department in a distressed state. His father and uncle had both died of heart attacks within weeks of each other, his father just two weeks earlier. Since then he had been getting episodes of chest pain exactly over his heart and he had been unable to sleep. At times he had been breathless. Arterial blood gases on air were as follows:

	Result	Normal range
pH	7.40	7.38–7.42
PCO_2	3.3 kPa	4.8–5.9
PO_2	14.9 kPa	10.6–13.3
Base excess	-8 mmol/l	-2 to +2

Interpretation: This patient has a normal pH but the PCO_2 is low, which should cause alkalosis. The reason the pH is normal is found in the base excess, which shows that there has been renal compensation. It seems that he must have been over-breathing for some time and the history is consistent with this. The PO_2 is high and this is consistent with the low PCO_2. This is a respiratory alkalosis with metabolic compensation.

SUMMARY

- ❏ The two main types of lung function defect are due to narrowed airways (obstructive) and small lungs (restrictive).
- ❏ Spirometry will distinguish between these two possibilities.
- ❏ A low FEV_1/VC (below 75% in the young) indicates airflow obstruction.
- ❏ A single peak flow reading may be difficult to interpret.
- ❏ Variable serial peak flows can confirm the diagnosis of asthma.
- ❏ Peak flows are useful in monitoring asthma severity.

- ❏ In chronic airways obstruction the VC may be low while the TLC may be high, reflecting gas trapping.

RECOMMENDED READING

Kinnear WJM (1997) Lung Function Tests. A Guide to their Interpretation. Nottingham University Press, Nottingham 1997.

ACKNOWLEDGEMENTS

The drawings are based on ones by Hugh Cummin.

Thoracic imaging

THE CHEST RADIOGRAPH

The chest radiograph (X-ray) is the cornerstone of thoracic imaging and should be considered an integral part of the respiratory examination. The chest radiograph is the most frequently requested radiological investigation worldwide.

To optimize the information obtained from a chest radiograph the patient should be standing erect with the anterior chest wall against the film cassette. The arms are abducted to rotate the scapulae away from the chest. The film is taken at maximal inspiration. The X-ray beam traverses the chest from back to front and is thus called the posteroanterior (PA) chest radiograph. If the patient is too ill to stand for a PA chest radiograph an anterior/posterior (AP) radiograph can be taken with the film cassette positioned behind the patient's back. In certain circumstances, where a third dimension is required to elucidate an abnormality on a PA radiograph, a lateral film can be obtained.

THE EVALUATION OF A CHEST RADIOGRAPH

The order in which a chest radiograph is scrutinized is unimportant. It is important, however, to have a fail-safe system that systematically examines all areas thoroughly. If there is a gross abnormality on a chest radiograph it is still important to carry out a thorough inspection to avoid missing other more subtle abnormalities. It is useful to know whether the patient has any old radiographs for comparison.

To aid interpretation it is important to note the age and racial origin of the patient when studying a chest radiograph. Hansell suggests the following order in which to scrutinize the film:

- ❏ Position of trachea.
- ❏ Mediastinal contour.
- ❏ Hilar shadows (position, outline, and density).
- ❏ Lungs (size, transradiancy, and collapse).
- ❏ Diaphragm (position and clarity).
- ❏ Ribs and soft tissues.

NORMAL ANATOMY ON A PLAIN RADIOGRAPH

Figure 15 shows a normal PA radiograph with labelling of the important structures. The mediastinal structures are superimposed on each other and are seen together as a unit. Further definition of the mediastinum can be seen on a CT scan and will be discussed later.

The cardiac silhouette should be clear and well defined. A loss of clarity to either border may suggest the presence of adjacent consolidation or collapse of the surrounding lung.

The trachea and main bronchi can be seen. The carina should be sharp. Splaying of the carina may indicate a subcarinal lymph node mass or an enlarged left atrium. The origins of the lobar bronchi can usually be seen through the mediastinal shadow.

The hila are composed of pulmonary arteries and veins. They should be the same size and density but the left hilum should lie between 0.5 and 1.5 cm above the right hilum.

The horizontal and oblique fissures separate the upper, middle, and lower lobes of the right lung. The oblique fissue is visible in 60% of individuals and is a useful landmark to assess for volume loss or collapse. The oblique fissure separates the upper and lower lobes of the left lung.

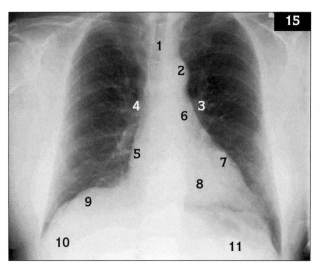

15 Normal PA chest radiograph. **1**, Trachea; **2**, Aortic arch; **3**, Left main pulmonary artery; **4**, Right main pulmonary artery; **5**, Right atrial border; **6**, Left atrial appendage; **7**, Left ventricular border; **8**, Right ventricle; **9**, Right dome diaphragm; **10**, Costophrenic angle; **11**, Gastric bubble

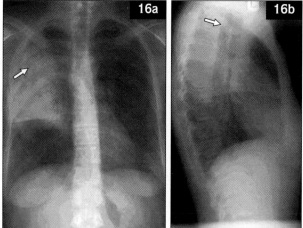

16 Air bronchograms in right upper lobe pneumonia: (**a**) PA and (**b**) lateral view

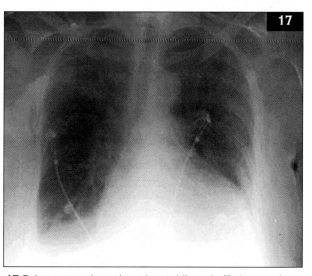

17 Pulmonary oedema; large heart, bilateral effusions, and perihilar shadowing

There should be a sharp line between the domes of the diaphragm and aerated lung. The diaphragm falls off sharply laterally to make an acute costophrenic angle. The right diaphragm is usually 2 cm higher than the left because of the presence of the liver below it.

SIGNS OF DISEASE ON THE CHEST RADIOGRAPH
Consolidation
This is where the distal air spaces – normally filled with air – are filled with something else, such as pus, water or blood. The abnormality commonly manifests as an area of increased shadowing that often contains an 'air bronchogram' and does not have a defined margin (**16**).

The causes of an air bronchogram are listed in *Table 7*. Consolidation is most commonly localized with infections such as pneumonia – 'lobar pneumonia'. A more diffuse pattern of air space infiltration is seen with water in the context of pulmonary oedema. Other features seen in pulmonary oedema to strengthen the diagnosis include pleural effusion (often bilateral), fluid in the fissures, and Kerly 'B' lines leading to the pleura (**17**). The cardiothoracic ratio may be increased (normally < 50%). In cases of pulmonary oedema the shadowing can often be seen to start at both hila and increase towards the periphery of the lung, the so-called 'bat's wing' shadowing.

While pulmonary oedema is the commonest cause

Table 7 Causes of an air bronchogram on a plain chest radiograph

❏ Consolidation
❏ Pulmonary oedema
❏ Blood
  Pulmonary haemorrhage
  Infarction
❏ Compression atelectasis (pleural effusion, pneumothorax)
❏ Fibrotic scarring (radiation fibrosis, bronchiectasis)
❏ Severe interstitial lung disease
❏ Neoplasms (bronchoalveolar cell carcinoma, lymphoma)

of bat's wing shadowing, other conditions such as *Pneumocystis* pneumonia (18) and lymphangitis carcinomatosis, may look similar.

Collapse

The terms collapse, loss of volume, and atelectasis are often used synonymously and can be applied to both partial and total lobar/lung collapse. Blockage of an airway causes loss of aeration, absorption of air, and deflation of the part of the lung supplied by that airway. This can occur from small sub-segmental areas to a whole lung. Postoperatively small areas of sub-segmental collapse are seen as linear, horizontal bands of atelectasis. Larger bronchi can be occluded by foreign bodies, mucous plugs, and tumours. It is important to recognize from the plain radiograph where the obstruction and collapse have occurred. The patterns accompanying individual lobar collapses are described below.

Right upper lobe collapse

There is elevation of the right hilum and the horizontal fissure. If the collapse is due to a small plug or small tumour the right upper lobe is seen as a density alongside the mediastinum. A juxtaphrenic peak may be visible owing to traction on a minor inferior fissure (19). If the collapse is due to a large tumour this can be seen as a mass within the collapse and gives rise to the 'Golden S' sign (20).

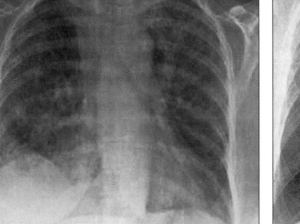

18 Pneumocystis pneumonia; dense perihilar infiltrates with sparing of apices and bases

19 Right upper lobe collapse; arrow marks juxtaphrenic peak

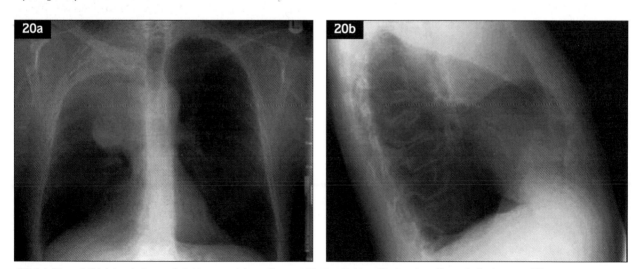

20 (**a**) PA and (**b**) lateral views of right upper lobe collapse with the Golden 'S' sign (*see* Case study 1, page 40)

Right middle lobe collapse
This can be very difficult to see on the PA radiograph but there may be subtle blurring of the right heart border. A lateral radiograph can be invaluable and show the oblique and horizontal fissures coming together to form a wedge anteriorly (**21**).

Right lower lobe collapse
The right hilum is pulled downwards and the right hemidiaphragm is obscured (**22**). The right heart border may remain sharp as this is next to the aerated right middle lobe. Again, as with middle lobe collapse, in subtle cases a lateral radiograph is very helpful as it may show increased opacification in the posterior portion of the lower spine.

Left upper lobe collapse
There is no horizontal fissure in the left lung so left upper lobe collapse is very different from that seen in the right lung. The collapsed upper lobe moves forward and upwards, pulling the left lower lobe upwards behind it. This is seen on a PA radiograph as a veil within the left hemithorax without any sharp margins (**23**). In some cases the apical segment of the left lower lobe may inflate into the lung apex giving the appearance of normally aerated left upper lobe in the apex.

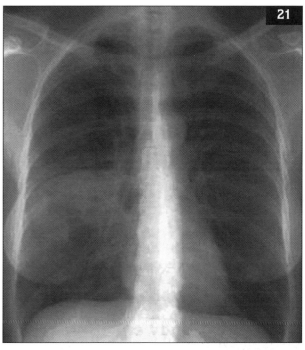

21 Right middle lobe collapse

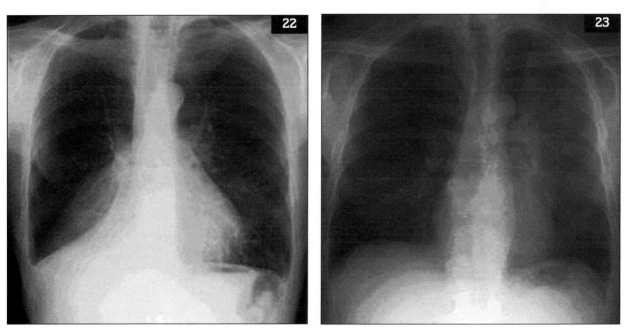

22 Right lower lobe collapse

23 Left upper lobe collapse

Left lower lobe collapse

As in right lower lobe collapse, the left hemidiaphragm is obscured, so here there is loss of some of the medial portion of the left hemidiaphragm (24). There may be a sharp linear density behind the left heart border or the heart border may appear bold and straight ('Sail' sign). The left hilum is pulled down.

Complete 'white-out'

The complete opacification of a whole hemithorax is due to either a complete lung collapse or a massive pleural effusion. The direction of shift in the mediastinum should clarify the diagnosis. Shift of the mediastinum towards the white-out suggests collapse (for example due to a main airway tumour or mucous plug) (25). Shift away from the white-out indicates a pleural effusion (see 62, page 92).

Masses and nodules

A pulmonary mass is a well defined opacity > 3 cm. A nodule has the same characteristics but is < 3 cm. A solitary pulmonary nodule (SPN) is one of the most common abnormalities discovered by chest radiography. On 95% of occasions it reflects one of the following:

❏ A malignant neoplasm (primary or metastatic).
❏ A granuloma (tuberculous or fungal).
❏ A benign tumour.

A more definitive list of causes of a SPN is shown in *Table 8*.

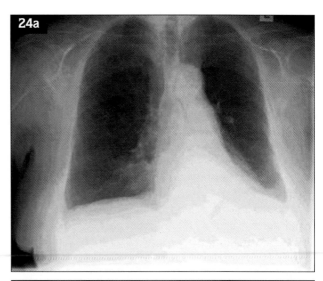

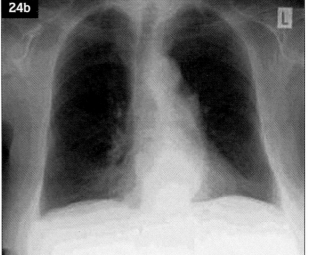

24 Left lower lobe collapse: (**a**), before and (**b**), after bronchoscopy

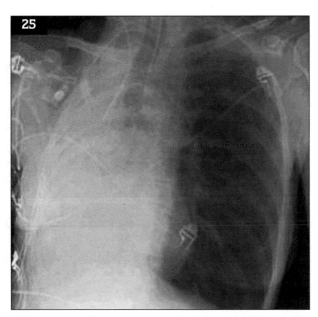

25 Right lung collapse – 'white-out' (*see* Case study 2, page 40)

Table 8 Differential diagnosis of a solitary pulmonary nodule

Neoplastic	Noninfective
Bronchial carcinoma	Rheumatoid arthritis
Metastasis	Wegener's granulomatosis
Carcinoid	Sarcoidosis
Lymphoma	Congenital atrioventricular malformations
	Lung cyst
Inflammatory	
	Miscellaneous
Infective	Pulmonary infarct
Granuloma (TB, fungal)	Lymph node
Pneumonia	Mucoid impaction
Lung abscess	
Hydatid cyst	

If a SPN is detected it is important to look at old radiographs to assess its possible growth. Features such as spiculation (a ragged edge), rapid growth, and cavitation suggest malignancy. Features such as calcification, slow growth, smooth edges, and a draining vein suggest a benign cause. The further investigation and management of the SPN is discussed in Chapter 5. Many of the features used to characterize malignancy in a SPN can also be applied to the assessment of a pulmonary mass, most of which are malignant. Their specific characteristics and management are discussed in Chapter 5.

Cavitation of a mass could indicate a squamous carcinoma. Cavitation is also known to occur in bacterial pneumonias such as those caused by *Staphylococcus* spp. and *Klebsiella* spp. Cavitation occurring in a mass can also rarely be seen with a resolving pulmonary infarct, especially in those occurring in the upper lobes. Long-standing cavities can be colonized by *Aspergillus* to give 'fungal balls' within an area of scarred lung.

Miliary pulmonary nodules

Miliary pulmonary nodules are usually < 2–5 mm in size. Classically on a chest radiograph these small nodules can be picked out individually with a pin. The commonest cause of miliary shadowing is tuberculosis (**26**). In this case the nodules are spread evenly from apex to base. Causes of miliary nodular shadowing are listed in *Box 4*.

OTHER TECHNIQUES IN THORACIC IMAGING
COMPUTED TOMOGRAPHY

Computed tomography (CT) is now established as an integral part of the work-up for specific patients with respiratory disease. CT generates cross-sectional images of the thorax that can be reconstructed in different planes to give a three-dimensional image of the chest (**27**). Newer CT scans are 'spiral' in nature meaning that the image is acquired in a spiral contiguous fashion. This significantly shortens the time taken to perform the scan and the radiation dosage is utilized to best effect. Indeed, the most recent CT scanners are able to acquire an image of the whole thorax within a single

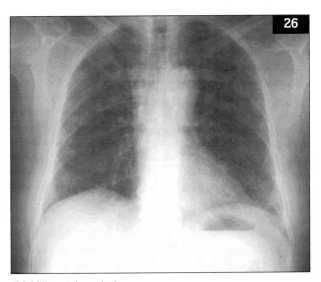

26 Miliary tuberculosis

> **BOX 4** Causes of miliary nodular shadowing
> (< 2–5 mm)
>
> ❏ Miliary tuberculosis.
> ❏ Fungal disease.
> ❏ Viral infection.
> ❏ Pneumoconiosis:
>   – Coal workers.
>   – Silicosis.
>   – Berylliosis.
> ❏ Sarcoidosis.
> ❏ Acute extrinsic allergic alveolitis.
> ❏ Metastases (carcinoma of the prostate).
> ❏ Histiocytosis X.

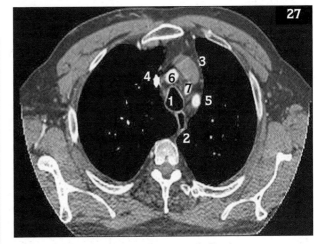

27 CT images of upper mediastinum: **1**, Trachea; **2**, Oesophagus; **3**, Lymphadenopathy; **4**, Superior vena cava; **5**, Left subclavian artery; **6**, Brachiocephalic artery; **7**, Left common carotid artery

breath-hold. CT can further image difficult areas, such as the mediastinum, to help with the staging of lung cancer and characterization of mediastinal masses. A CT pulmonary angiogram (CT-PA) can be used to detect central and segmental pulmonary emboli without the need for more invasive angiography (**28**). The use of CT for the staging of a SPN and in lung cancer has already been described. Finer CT cuts of 1 mm (vs. 10 mm for lung cancer staging) are used to assess for diffuse parenchymal lung disease (see Chapter 8, page 80). Indications for a CT scan of the thorax are listed in *Box 5*.

ULTRASOUND

The main use for ultrasound of the chest is in the localization and characterization of a pleural effusion. It can also be used to guide percutaneous drainage of effusions and needle biopsies of abnormal pleural or lung masses abutting the pleura.

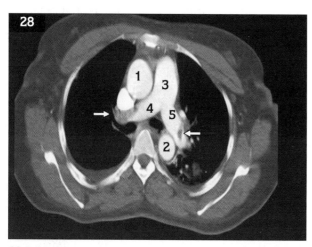

28 Pulmonary emboli (arrowed) in main pulmonary arteries in a CT pulmonary angiogram: **1**, Ascending aorta; **2**, Descending aorta; **3**, Main pulmonary artery; **4**, Right pulmonary artery; **5**, Left pulmonary artery

VENTILATION–PERFUSION (VQ) SCANNING

The patient inhales an inert gas with an ultra-short half-life (e.g. Krypton) to assess ventilation and this is compared to images obtained from the injection of radiolabelled technetium. The thorax is scanned using gamma rays. Areas of unmatched perfusion compared to ventilation may be suggestive of pulmonary embolic disease (**29**). In patients with lung disease, such as asthma or COPD, the perfusion scan similarly shows perfusion defects. However, in these cases the perfusion defects reflect hypoxic vasoconstriction in an area of diminished ventilation – so-called matched ventilation/perfusion defects. A VQ scan must be interpreted in the light of a recent chest radiograph and the clinical history. VQ scanning can also be used to assess patients with COPD before lung cancer surgery.

MAGNETIC RESONANCE IMAGING (MRI)

In magnetic resonance imaging (MRI) a powerful magnet generates a magnetic field and a very small percentage of hydrogen atoms within the body will align with this field. Radio wave pulses are broadcast towards the aligned hydrogen atoms in tissues of interest, which return a signal of their own. The subtly differing characteristics of that signal from different tissues enable MRI to differentiate between various organs. There is no ionizing radiation involved in MRI, and there have been no documented significant side-effects of the magnetic fields and radio waves used on the human body to date.

MRI has become the modality of choice in many diagnostic studies of the head, spine, and joints. It can also provide detailed pictures of tissues within the chest cavity, without obstruction by overlying bone. It is most commonly used to clarify findings from previous radiographs or CT scans where cystic/mass-like lesions need further delineation. MRI can show the structures of the chest from multiple planes and can, therefore, be

---

BOX 5 Indications for a computed tomography (CT) scan of the thorax

10 mm spiral CT
❏ Suspected or proven lung cancer for staging (must include liver and adrenal glands and IV contrast to assess lymph nodes).
❏ Evaluation of a solitary nodule.
❏ Further evaluation of an abnormal hilum or mediastinal shadow.
❏ Pleural disease.

High-resolution CT (HRCT)
❏ Patients with suspected diffuse parenchymal lung disease.
❏ Staging patients with COPD/emphysema.
CT-PA
❏ Suspected pulmonary embolism.
Intervention
❏ Percutaneous needle biopsy.
❏ Positioning of a difficult chest drain.

very useful for assessing tumour invasion into the chest wall or mediastinum and providing information for the more accurate staging of tumours in the chest cavity.

Currently, MRI is not routinely valuable in the evaluation of subtle changes of the lung tissue since the lungs contain mostly air and are difficult to image. However, inhaled radiolabelled helium has been used to assess functional regional lung diffusion in research studies. This may be an exciting tool in the future to give a more accurate early assessment of emphysema.

POSITRON EMISSION TOMOGRAPHY

Positron emission tomography (PET) measures glucose uptake into tissue following the administration of radiolabelled glucose (fluorodeoxyglucose, FDG) into the patient. Areas of high metabolic activity take up the glucose and release positrons which can be detected by a gamma camera. The radiation dose of a PET scan is equivalent to that from a CT scan. Organs, such as the heart and the brain, have a high metabolic state and therefore are very FDG-avid and appear black ('hot') on the scan. Most types of tumour and areas of acute inflammation in the body are also FDG-avid and will give a positive scan. Functional imaging by PET complements and enhances the staging and detection of tumours by imaging modalities (radiography, CT, and MRI) which demonstrate anatomical changes. More recent PET scanners are dual PET/CT scans and can co-register images so PET hot-spots can be correlated with the anatomical area simultaneously. Most tumours have an increased requirement for glucose compared to that of normal tissue. Therefore, PET scanning can allow detection of primary tumours and metastases. Tumours which grow slowly may be negative on PET scanning, for example bronchoalveolar cell carcinoma. As the brain has a high requirement for glucose and is positive in normals it is difficult to identify primary or secondary brain tumours by this method. However, PET is very useful for detecting extrathoracic metastases in bone and adrenal glands. Inflammatory conditions which increase turnover of glucose will also be hot on PET scanning, e.g. tuberculosis and sarcoidosis. Therefore, PET has a low specificity but a very high sensitivity for cancers. PET cannot replace conventional imaging and tissue confirmation of primary tumours still needs to be made. Other investigational uses of PET scanning in respiratory medicine include the assessment of particle distribution throughout the lung following inhaled medication.

SUMMARY

❏ The PA chest radiograph is an excellent tool for respiratory imaging.

❏ A lateral radiograph can help to delineate lobar collapse.

❏ Always ask the patient about the availability of any previous radiographs for comparison.

❏ CT scanning of the thorax is essential in lung cancer staging and for further evaluation of difficult radiographs.

❏ MRI of the thorax is not routine.

❏ PET scanning is a further valuable tool in the staging of intrathoracic malignancy.

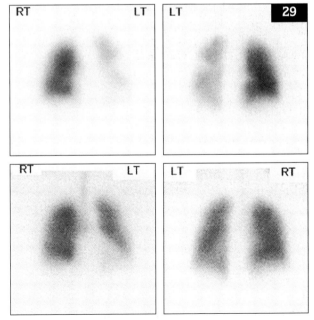

29 Ventilation–perfusion scan showing reduced perfusion to left lung with preserved ventilation

CASE STUDIES

CASE STUDY 1

Mr JD, a 60-year-old life-long smoker, presented with shortness of breath and a red swollen face. His chest radiograph is shown on page 34 (**20**). A right upper lobe lung cancer was suspected with superior vena cava obstruction (SVCO). This was confirmed on venography and a stent was placed *in situ* (see **38b**). At bronchoscopy a fleshy tumour was found occluding the right upper lobe bronchus. This was found to be a small cell carcinoma. Following chemotherapy the mass was significantly smaller and the right upper lobe collapse less marked (**30**). He was no longer short of breath.

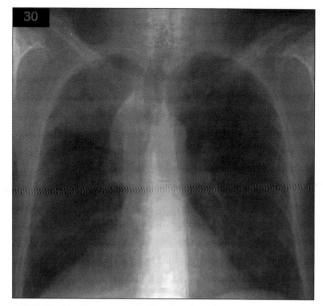

30 Patient in Case study 1 after treatment

CASE STUDY 2

Mrs JP, a 70-year-old woman, was admitted straight to ITU from the emergency department for respiratory failure. Her chest radiograph is shown on page 36 (**25**). She was immediately ventilated. At bronchoscopy a large mucous plug was found occluding her right main bronchus. This was successfully removed using high-flow suction and warm saline lavage through the bronchoscope. Her chest radiograph after bronchoscopy is shown (**31**). Further investigations showed Mrs JP to have allergic bronchopulmonary aspergillosis (see Chapter 7, page 70).

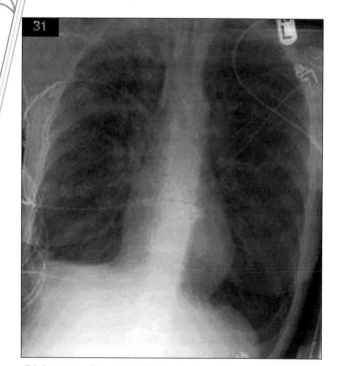

31 Patient in Case study 2 after treatment

SECTION B: DISEASES AND DISORDERS OF THE RESPIRATORY SYSTEM

Chapter 5
LUNG CANCER (AND OTHER INTRATHORACIC MALIGNANCY)

Chapter 6
CHRONIC OBSTRUCTIVE PULMONARY DISEASE

Chapter 7
ASTHMA

Chapter 8
DIFFUSE PARENCHYMAL (INTERSTITIAL) LUNG DISEASE

Chapter 9
PLEURAL DISEASES

Chapter 10
INFECTIONS OF THE RESPIRATORY TRACT

Chapter 11
SUPPURATIVE LUNG CONDITIONS

Chapter 12
SLEEP-RELATED BREATHING DISORDERS

Chapter 13
RESPIRATORY FAILURE

Chapter 14
PULMONARY VASCULAR PROBLEMS

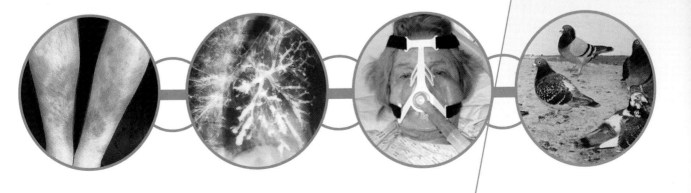

Chapter 5 Lung cancer (and other intrathoracic malignancy)

INTRODUCTION

Lung cancer (bronchial carcinoma) is the commonest cancer in the Western world and is the most lethal cancer. In the UK it is the commonest cancer in men and the third commonest cancer in women. Death due to lung cancer is the third commonest cause of death after heart disease and pneumonia. 34,000 people died of lung cancer in 1999. It has always been the commonest cause of cancer death in men but in 2001 it also became the commonest cause of cancer death in women, overtaking breast cancer. There are more deaths in the UK from lung cancer than from breast, colon, prostate, and cervical cancer put together. Lung cancer was a rare disease at the start of the 20th century but now, following exposure to aetiological agents and with an increasing lifespan, it has become the commonest and most lethal cancer.

By far the most common aetiological agent associated with the development of lung cancer is cigarette smoking, accounting for approximately 90% of all lung cancer cases. This association was brought to the fore by Doll and colleagues in the landmark British doctors' study in the 1950s that showed the association between number of cigarettes smoked and the development of lung cancer (32).

Passive smoking (the inhalation of other people's smoke by nonsmokers) increases the risk of lung cancer by a factor of 1.5. There are other causes of lung cancer, including exposure to asbestos, arsenic, chromates, nickel, polycyclic aromatic hydrocarbons, and radon. A smoker who has been exposed to asbestos has a lung cancer risk more than 100 times a nonsmoker who has never come across asbestos. Outdoor air pollution is also thought to contribute to the development of lung cancer and this is shown by the burden of lung cancer in urbanized areas. In densely populated cities in China cooking fumes from rapeseed and linseed oils used for cooking in small kitchens are thought to play an increasing role in the development of lung cancer in nonsmoking women.

Cigarette smoke and other carcinogens, helped by host factors such as a shift to metabolic activation from detoxification, cause the formation of DNA adducts. If these adducts are repaired then normal DNA is restored; if left they can develop into a lung cancer (33).

As smoking is the major cause of lung cancer smoking cessation is very important. Rates of lung cancer lag behind smoking trends by 29 years (approximately), emphasizing the importance of smoking cessation by young people as soon as possible. The likelihood of lung cancer decreases amongst those who no longer smoke compared to those who continue. As the period of abstinence increases, the risk of lung cancer decreases (*Table 9*).

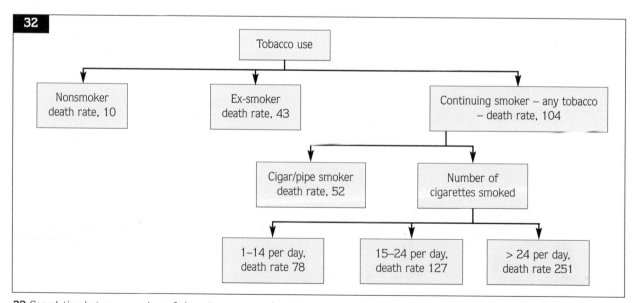

32 Correlation between number of cigarettes consumed and lung cancer risk (from Doll's and Hill's Doctors' study, 1956); death rates per 100,000 population

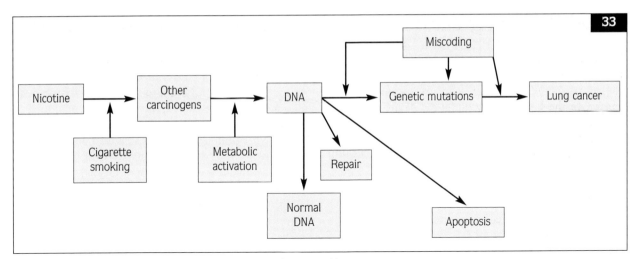

33 Putative pathway from nicotine addiction to the development of lung cancer

Table 9 Risk of lung cancer decreases with increasing periods of abstinence

Years since smoked	Cigarettes smoked per day				Total ex-smokers
	1–9	10–20	21–39	> 40	
< 5	7.6	12.5	20.6	26.9	16.1
5–9	3.6	5.1	11.5	13.6	7.8
10–19	2.2	4.3	6.8	7.8	5.1
20–29	1.7	3.3	3.4	5.9	3.3
30–39	0.5	2.1	2.8	4.5	2.0
> 40	1.1	1.6	1.8	2.3	1.5

CELL TYPES

Lung cancer is divided into nonsmall cell carcinoma (NSCLC) and small cell carcinoma, based on the morphological characteristics of the tumour cells and their immunophenotyping. In making a diagnosis of lung cancer it is imperative to know the cell type, as the prognosis and treatment for each type can be very different. Department of Health guidelines state that over 85% of patients with suspected lung cancer should have a confirmed tissue diagnosis.

NONSMALL-CELL CARCINOMA (NSCLC)

NSCLC make up over 70% of all lung cancer diagnoses. However, over the last few years the frequency of certain histological NSCLC sub-types has been changing. There has been a gradual decrease in the prevalence of squamous (epidermoid) cell carcinoma and an increase in adenocarcinoma. Adenocarcinoma now accounts for 50% of all NSCLC with squamous cell carcinoma comprising 35%, large cell carcinoma comprising 10%, and alveolar cell carcinoma contributing 5%. Some of this change is thought to be due to a change in cigarette composition from high-yield to low-yield brands with filters. The filter cigarette smoker needs a deeper inhalation and this allows smoke particles and carcinogens to reach the periphery of the lung. The relative risks of smokers developing different lung cancer cell types are shown in *Table 10*.

Adenocarcinoma

Adenocarcinoma usually arises in the periphery of the lung from mucous glands in the small bronchi. Adenocarcinoma has an intermediate doubling time (approximately 60–80 days). It may present as a

Table 10 Relative risk for smokers for types of tumour

Tumour type	Relative risk in smokers (RR = 1 for nonsmokers)
Small cell	14
Squamous cell	8
Large cell	7
Adenocarcinoma	4

solitary pulmonary nodule (SPN) (70%, 34), as an area of mass-like consolidation (20%) or as a pleural effusion (10%). This is the commonest cancer type in association with occupational lung disease and scar tissue – and the cancer least associated with cigarette consumption. To confirm a diagnosis of primary lung adenocarcinoma immunophenotyping is often required to exclude adenocarcinoma metastases from other common adenocarcinomas, such as breast, colon, prostate, and renal. Thyroid transcription factor (TTF-1) expression is the most important marker for this. Adenocarcinomas often invade locally and have often metastasized before presentation.

Squamous cell carcinoma

Squamous cell carcinoma arises from the epithelium of the main bronchi and is likely to present with symptoms of airway obstruction or haemoptysis. Occasionally solitary masses attributable to squamous cell carcinoma can cavitate (35). A cavity wall thickness of > 15 mm is thought to be indicative of malignancy. Squamous cell carcinoma has the longest cell doubling time of over 90 days. The cells are usually well differentiated and local spread is more common than distant metastases.

Large cell carcinoma

Large cell carcinoma is a poorly differentiated type of NSCLC that metastasizes early and has a poor prognosis.

Bronchoalveolar cell carcinoma

Bronchoalveolar cell carcinoma (also called alveolar cell carcinoma) is a well differentiated subtype of adenocarcinoma. It may present as a SPN or as diffuse consolidation. In the form of diffuse consolidation the patient may present with copious amounts of white sputum and a cytological diagnosis can be made from this.

SMALL-CELL CARCINOMA

Small-cell or oat cell carcinoma makes up the remaining 20–30% of lung cancers. It is the cancer most associated with smoking. It arises from endocrine cells that are part of the amine precursor uptake and decarboxylation (APUD) system. These cells can secrete many polypeptides that can cause a variety of paraneoplastic syndromes (see later). Small-cell carcinoma has the fastest doubling time of all lung cancer types and is often a systemic disease at presentation. The high cell turnover does mean, however, that small cell carcinoma can respond very well, at least initially, to high-dose chemotherapy.

THE PATIENT WITH SUSPECTED LUNG CANCER

HISTORY AND EXAMINATION

From the introduction above it can seen how important it is to get a good, clear smoking and occupational history. It is important to determine any lung cancer related symptoms (*Table 11*) and to assess the patient's respiratory reserve and performance status (*Table 12*).

There may be no abnormal physical signs. Local tumour growth, invasion or obstruction, growth in local nodes, growth in metastatic sites, and remote effects (paraneoplastic) can cause signs and symptoms. Only 15% of lung cancer is detected while the patients are asymptomatic. The remainder tend to present with advanced, symptomatic disease. It is important to look for clubbing (most often with NSCLC rather than small-cell carcinoma) (36) and local lymph node spread (supraclavicular and axillary). Endobronchial disease may give signs of a fixed expiratory monophonic wheeze, stridor or of an obstructive pneumonia and lobar collapse. Symptoms and signs of peripheral tumour growth are inspiratory pain, due to pleural infiltration/pleural fluid or chest wall infiltration. Abdominal examination may reveal an enlarged liver.

Bronchial carcinoma may spread directly to invade local structures and cause local signs. A Pancoast's tumour sits in the superior sulcus (lung apex) (37) and can invade the brachial plexus (C8, T1) causing severe pain in the affected dermatomes. If the sympathetic ganglion is also involved the patient may have a Horner's syndrome. Tumours arising in the hilar regions may spread to invade the recurrent laryngeal nerve, causing hoarseness. Direct tumour invasion of the phrenic nerve causes ipsilateral paralysis. Tumours can invade other local structures, such as the pericardium (pericardial effusion and tamponade), the oesophagus (dysphagia), and the superior vena cava (SVC). SVC obstruction (SVCO) can occur in up to 10% of patients with lung cancer and is most often caused by small-cell carcinoma. Symptoms are early morning facial plethora and headaches, facial and upper limb oedema, and distended neck and chest wall veins. Treatment should be either immediate radiotherapy or the insertion of a stent under radiological control (38).

Lung cancers most commonly spread to bone (pain, pathological fractures, and hypercalcemia), brain (headaches, fits, and focal neurological signs), liver (hepatomegaly, pain, and abnormal liver function tests), and adrenal glands (very rarely symptomatic).

Nonmetastatic extrapulmonary manifestations of lung cancer and associated paraneoplastic syndromes

34 Adeno-carcinoma in the 2nd R intercostal space presenting as a solitary pulmonary nodule

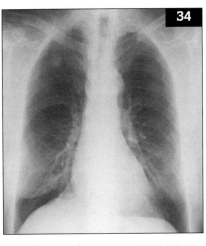

Table 11 The frequencies of the most common presenting symptoms and signs of lung cancer

Symptoms and signs	Range of frequency (%)
Cough	10–75
Weight loss	0–68
Dyspnoea	5–60
Chest pain	20–50
Haemoptysis	6–35
Bone pain	6–25
Clubbing	0–20
Weakness	0–10
Superior vena cava obstruction	0–10
Stridor	0–4
Dysphagia	0–2

35 Cavitating squamous cell carcinoma

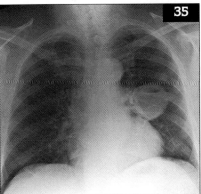

Table 12 WHO performance scale

Grade	Description
0	Fully active, can carry out all functions without restriction
1	Restricted in strenuous activity; ambulatory, can carry out light work, e.g. office work
2	Ambulatory and capable of self-care but unable to carry out work activities. Up and about for more than 50% of waking hours
3	Capable of limited self-care; confined to bed/chair for more than 50% of waking hours
4	Completely disabled. Confined to bed/chair

36 Digital clubbing

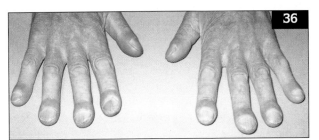

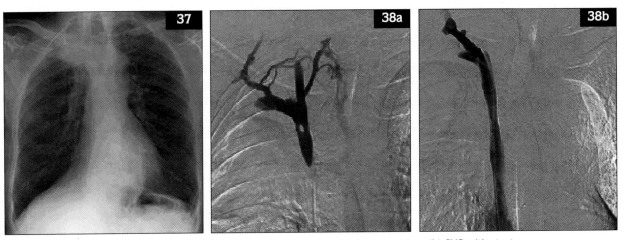

37 Pancoast's tumour in the lung apex

38 (**a**) Superior vena cava (SVC) obstruction; (**b**) SVC with stent

are shown in *Table 13*. Hypertrophic osteoarthropathy (HOA) manifests as arthropathy, periostitis, and finger clubbing, and is usually associated with adenocarcinoma. It most commonly affects the distal ends of the long bones (**39**). It is thought to be caused by an unknown humoral factor, and transforming growth factor-beta (TGF-β) has been postulated. Surgical removal or radical radiotherapy to the tumour causes spontaneous regression of the HOA.

Hyponatreamia is the commonest endocrine abnormality in lung cancer. Any lung cancer or pneumonia can cause the syndrome of inappropriate antidiuretic hormone secretion (SIADH). However small cell lung cancer cells can also directly secrete antidiuretic hormone (ADH). This ADH binds to collecting duct receptors, leading to free water retention which results in a hypo-osmolar plasma with inappropriate hyperosmolarity in urine. Hypercalcaemia can be either humoral or osteolytic. Humoral hypercalcaemia is related to the secretion of parathyroid-like hormone related peptide (PTHrP) by squamous cell carcinomas; this binds to parathyroid hormone (PTH) receptors, causing increased bone reabsorption, decreased bone formation, and increased tubular reabsorption. Osteolytic hypercalcaemia can occur by direct invasion of bone by metastatic tumours. Hyperthyroidism, gynaecomastia, and disorders of glucose metabolism are rarely encountered.

INVESTIGATIONS

In clinic the patient should have spirometry and oximetry performed to assess suitability for invasive investigations and surgery and to assess the extent of respiratory co-morbidity. Blood tests should be taken for full blood count, coagulation studies (if biopsies are to be performed), electrolytes, and bone and liver biochemistry. Lung tumour markers, such as squamous cell antigen (SCA) and neurone specific enolase (NSE) for small-cell carcinoma, can be used to follow up response to treatment but should not be used as screening tools.

RADIOLOGICAL INVESTIGATIONS

Most symptomatic lung cancers are visible on a plain chest radiograph. Occasionally small asymptomatic tumours > 1 cm can be seen on radiographs taken routinely for another purpose (e.g. pre-operation). A normal chest radiograph in the presence of haemoptysis or monophonic wheeze does not exclude a lung cancer. Lung cancers arising in the main airways may manifest on the radiograph as a hilar mass (**40**) or a lobar collapse (see Chapter 4, page 34). The mediastinum may be widened by hilar nodes (**41**).

In order to obtain a more detailed assessment of the position of the tumour, to plan appropriate investigation and to complete staging, a computed axial tomography (CT) scan is performed. The scan covers the lung apices to the adrenal glands to identify metastases. Intravenous contrast is given to enable a full assessment of hilar and mediastinal lymph nodes. For central lesions or areas of consolidative tumour a bronchoscopy is the diagnostic modality of choice. For peripheral tumours a transthoracic needle aspiration biopsy (TNAB) is performed.

BRONCHOSCOPY

Fibre-optic bronchoscopy is a day-case procedure performed under conscious sedation. The operator can assess the extent of the tumour as well as making an assessment with regards to suitability for surgical resection. Tissue samples can be taken via the bronchoscope with biopsy forceps, with a cytological brush, and with saline lavage. Combining all three diagnostic modalities increases the diagnostic rate to > 85%.

TRANSTHORACIC NEEDLE ASPIRATION BIOPSY (TNAB)

TNAB is performed under either direct CT vision or ultrasound. The operator localizes the lesion with the imaging modality of choice, anaesthetizes the skin and passes a fine needle or cutting (biopsy) needle into the centre of the lesion. The diagnostic yield can be up to 90%, especially with an on-site cytopathologist to evaluate the adequacy of the sample. There is an iatrogenic pneumothorax rate of up to 20%. Patients should only undergo a TNAB if they are able to withstand a significant pneumothorax.

SPUTUM CYTOLOGY

Central airway tumours may shed malignant cells into sputum and be identified in up to 60% of cases. Ideally three early morning sputum samples should be obtained. Peripheral lesions are less likely to yield a positive sputum result.

PLEURAL EFFUSION CYTOLOGY

Patients with pleural effusions should have 50 mls of fluid aspirated in aseptic fashion and this should be sent for cytological diagnosis. If this is nondiagnostic the patient may require direct examination of the pleura with a thoracoscope under general anaesthetic, or a percutaneous pleural biopsy, either using an Abrams pleural biopsy needle or under CT guidance.

Table 13 Nonmetastatic extrapulmonary manifestations of lung cancer and associated para-neoplastic syndromes

Type	Signs	Frequency
Skeletal	Clubbing	30% (NSCLC > small-cell)
	Hypertrophic osteoarthropathy	10% (NSCLC > small-cell)
Metabolic	Weight loss and anorexia	Universal at some time
	Fever	Universal at some time
	Lethargy	Universal at some time
Endocrine	Low sodium, SIADH	10–15%
	Hypercalcaemia	15%
	Ectopic ACTH	< 5% small-cell
Neurological	Encephalopathy	2–15%
	Myelopathy	2–15%
	Peripheral neuropathy	2–15%
	Muscular disorders (Eaton–Lambert syndrome with small-cell)	2–15%
Haematological	Anaemia	0–10%
	Leucocytosis; eosinophilia	0–10%
	Leukaemoid reaction	0–10%
	Thrombocytosis	0–10%
	Disseminated intravascular coagulation	0–10%
Collagen/vascular	Dermatomyositis	0–5%
	Polymyositis	0–5%
	Vasculitis	0–5%
Dermatological	Erythema multiforme	0–5%
	Erythema gyratum repens	0–5%
	Acanthosis nigricans	0–5%

ACTH, adrenocorticotropic hormone; NSCLC, nonsmall-cell carcinoma; SIADH, syndrome of inappropriate antidiuretic hormone secretion

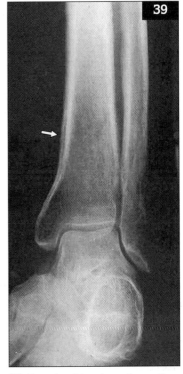

39 Hypertrophic osteoarthropathy with periosteal new bone formation (arrow)

40 Right hilar mass

41 Mediastinal and hilar lymph node enlargement

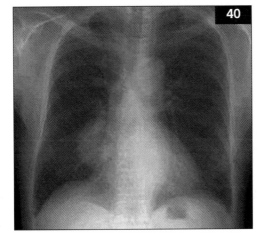

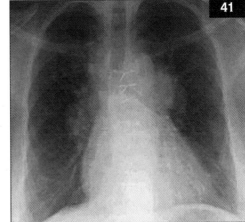

STAGING FOR LUNG CANCER

Further extrathoracic staging is only requested if there are specific patient symptoms. Bone pain should lead to a bone scan, and headaches or focal neurology to a CT scan of the brain. There is no evidence that performing these investigations in the absence of symptoms improves management. Once the histological type is known and the staging is complete the patient should be discussed in a meeting of the multi-disciplinary team (MDT) which includes chest physicians, radiologists, pathologists, thoracic surgeons, oncologists, and palliative care physicians. The patient's performance status, lung function and clinical stage (*Tables 14* and *15*, page 48) are used to make an appropriate treatment plan. If there are mediastinal lymph nodes on the CT scan > 1 cm in length further assessment of the mediastinum is required. This could be via a mediastinoscopy or with a PET scan. Fluorodeoxyglucose positron emission tomography (FDG-PET) has been shown to have a high negative predicative value for mediastinal staging pre-operatively. The FDG is taken up preferentially by dividing tumour cells rather than inflammatory cells. A negative PET scan is 95% correct for negative mediastinal nodes and the patient can be advised to proceed to surgery. As other inflammatory conditions, such as tuberculosis and sarcoid, can take up FDG, a positive PET scan requires further invasive investigation before the patient is deemed unsuitable for surgery.

TREATMENT

SURGERY

Surgical resection represents the only treatment that is likely to offer the NSCLC patient the possibility of long-term survival of over 5 years. Surgery for small-cell carcinoma is unlikely to be curative. Patients with tumours of stage IIb or lower are amenable to surgery if their FEV_1 is > 1.5 l for a lobectomy or 2.0 l for a pneumonectomy. For borderline cases further assessment with shuttle tests (see Chapter 4, page 24) and VQ scanning can help to predict postoperative morbidity. Only 5–10% patients in the UK are referred for surgical resection. With the advent of the MDT it is hoped that this figure will be nearer 15% as more patients are discussed with the surgeons.

However, it is sadly the case that, for whatever reason, most patients present to their GP/hospital with advanced lung cancer that is inoperable at presentation.

RADIOTHERAPY

Radiotherapy can be given in the radical (curative) setting or for symptom control (palliative). Radical radiotherapy can be given to patients with localized NSCLC who are medically unfit for surgery or who do not want surgery. Squamous cell carcinomas are generally more radiosensitive than adenocarcinomas. Radical radiotherapy is now mapped in 3-D on special CT scans to minimize damage to normal lung and surrounding structures. Up to 60 Gray is given in 4–6-week courses. Five-year survival is not as good as with surgery. A recent study has shown that giving the radiotherapy three times a day for a continuous period of 12 days (including weekends) has improved survival compared to the standard once daily, 5 days a week, treatment. Unfortunately, lack of resources means that this is not standard treatment in the UK.

Radiotherapy can be given after surgery if the resection margins are positive or N3 nodes were found at operation. This prevents local disease relapse but does not improve survival. There is no role for pre-operative radiotherapy.

Table 14 'TNM' classification		
Primary tumour (**T**)	T0	None evident
	T1	< 3 cm in lobar/distal airway
	T2	> 3 cm and > 2 cm from carina Obstructive pneumonia
	T3	Involves the chest wall, diaphragm, pleura < 2 cm from carina
	T4	Invades mediastinum, heart, great vessels Malignant effusion
Regional nodes (**N**)	N0	None
	N1	Peribronchial and/or ipsilateral hilum
	N2	Ipsilateral mediastinum or subcarinal
	N3	Contralateral mediastinum/hilum, supraclavicular
Distant metastases (**M**)	M0	None
	M1	Present

Table 15 The international staging system for lung cancer

TNM			New classification	5-year survival (%)
T1	N0	M0	Ia	61
T2	N0	M0	Ib	38
T1	N1	M0	IIa	34
T2	N1	M0	IIb	24
T3	N0	M0	IIb	22
T3	N1	M0	IIIa	9
T1–3	N2	M0	IIIa	13
T4	N0–-2	M0	IIIb	7
T1–4	N3	M0	IIIb	3
M1 or several nodules in different lobes			IV	1

CF Mountain. *Chest* 1997;**111**:1710–1717.

Palliative radiotherapy can be very effective at managing symptoms, such as cough or haemoptysis secondary to endobronchial disease. Palliative doses of radiotherapy are much lower (i.e. < 20 Gray) and given over a shorter course. Palliative treatment is also effective for SVCO and single painful bone secondaries. Disease in the brain and spinal cord can also be treated but effects are less impressive.

Radiotherapy can also be delivered directly into the bronchus to treat endoluminal compression or haemoptysis. This is done as an outpatient treatment using a standard flexible bronchoscope. Usually only one treatment dose is given.

CHEMOTHERAPY

Small-cell lung cancer

Chemotherapy is the treatment of choice for this disease as the rapid cell turnover enables the cellular

DNA to incorporate cytotoxic drugs. If left untreated death occurs within 6 weeks. The survival of patients with small-cell carcinoma has increased gradually over the last decade. Very good tumour responses can be seen with initial chemotherapy, although relapse is very common. Most combinations would include cyclophosphamide, doxorubicin, and vincristine, followed by cisplatin and etoposide. This regimen is given every 3 weeks for up to six cycles. Eighty percent of patients will have a response with this regimen as measured by reduction in tumour size and 70% of patients will have an improvement in their symptom score. Radiotherapy can be given after chemotherapy to treat mediastinal lymph node disease and to prevent disease from spreading to the brain.

Nonsmall-cell carcinoma

Approximately 80% of patients with NSCLC present with advanced disease and are not suitable for surgery or radical radiotherapy. Previously only 1–20% of these patients would receive palliative chemotherapy, as there was little evidence that chemotherapy extended survival. This idea began to change in 2000 when it was shown that platinum-based chemotherapy significantly improves both symptom control and quality of life. In July 2001 the UK National Institute for Clinical Excellence (NICE) reviewed the role of chemotherapy in NSCLC. NICE concluded that chemotherapy for NSCLC should be considered in all patients who have advanced disease (stages III and IV) and of good performance status (WHO performance score 0–2, *Table 12*, page 45). They recommended that a platinum-based agent should be combined with one of gemcitabine, vinorelbine or paclitaxel, to offer the most clinically and cost-effective approach. All of these agents can be given as outpatient-based treatment and have significantly fewer distressing side-effects such as hair loss. Not only are these agents well tolerated, but they can offer effective symptom control and have been shown in clinical trials to extend median survival from 5 to 9 months on average.

Chemotherapy and surgery

There is no convincing evidence that chemotherapy after surgery (whether complete or incomplete surgical resection), given in the adjuvant setting, prolongs survival.

Two small studies in 1994 suggested a survival benefit for patients with IIIa NSCLC if they received chemotherapy pre-operatively (neo-adjuvant chemotherapy). The authors postulated that chemotherapy in this setting treated any micrometastases already circulating. There was an increase in postoperative morbidity in the chemotherapy group and a very small number of patients progressed while on chemotherapy. The concept of neo-adjuvant chemotherapy for any stage patient with NSCLC being considered for surgery is the subject of an ongoing randomized Medical Research Council (MRC) study, and any such patient should be offered randomization into MRC LU22.

LUNG CANCER PREVENTION

The most important aspect of lung cancer prevention is smoking cessation and avoidance (i.e. preventing young children and teenagers from smoking). It is hoped that the banning of all cigarette advertising from 2003 will help towards this. For people already addicted to nicotine, general practitioners are now able to prescribe nicotine replacement therapy (NRT). NRT can also be prescribed for NHS hospital inpatients. It is important to remember that > 40% of patients on medical wards and 60% on vascular wards are smokers. This 'captive audience' should be offered smoking cessation advice and NRT. It is the health care professional's role to 'ask, advise, and assist' all patients in the hospital setting who smoke to address and treat their addiction (see *Table 17*, page 55).

There is currently no evidence that primary chemoprevention with oral vitamins and/or antioxidants reduces the incidence of lung cancer.

LUNG CANCER SCREENING

The published evidence does not support the use of the plain chest radiograph with or without sputum cytology for the early detection of lung cancer. Recent studies have focused on the use of low-dose CT (LDCT) screening of high-risk patients. Early results have suggested that lung cancer can be detected at an early stage (< 1 cm) and can be resected. There are, however, concerns that LDCT may detect slow-growing lung cancers that are not likely to kill the patient in their lifetime and patients may be subjected to an unnecessary thoracotomy. Furthermore, screening is often associated with a high false positive rate – that is, the detection of a significant number of lesions needing investigation but not subsequently being shown to be a cancer. To date the LDCT studies have not shown a reduction in disease-specific mortality due to early detection. Currently there are several US and European-wide LDCT randomized trials, and physicians and patients should be advised to enter these trials rather than requesting a stand-alone LDCT.

CASE STUDY

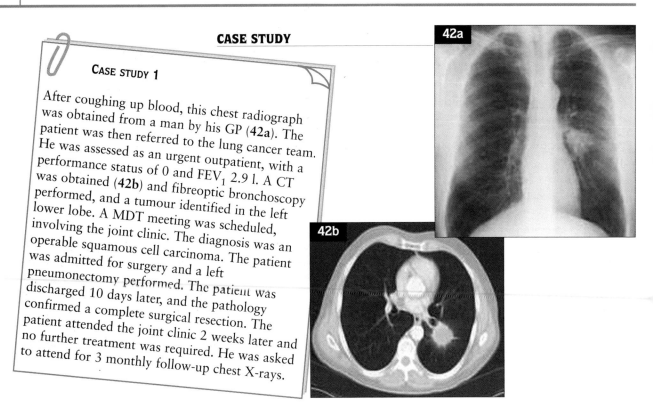

CASE STUDY 1

After coughing up blood, this chest radiograph was obtained from a man by his GP (**42a**). The patient was then referred to the lung cancer team. He was assessed as an urgent outpatient, with a performance status of 0 and FEV_1 2.9 l. A CT was obtained (**42b**) and fibreoptic bronchoscopy performed, and a tumour identified in the left lower lobe. A MDT meeting was scheduled, involving the joint clinic. The diagnosis was an operable squamous cell carcinoma. The patient was admitted for surgery and a left pneumonectomy performed. The patient was discharged 10 days later, and the pathology confirmed a complete surgical resection. The patient attended the joint clinic 2 weeks later and no further treatment was required. He was asked to attend for 3 monthly follow-up chest X-rays.

CARCINOID TUMOURS

Carcinoid tumours often present as single nodules or small masses. They are not associated with smoking and often occur in younger people than does lung cancer. These tumours used to be classified as benign but can in some instances (10%) become malignant and spread to local and regional nodes. Patients most commonly present with cough and haemoptysis. Less than 20% of lung carcinoids produce the classic carcinoid syndrome of flushing, cramps, and diarrhoea. The majority of lesions are within the main bronchi and can be seen and sampled at bronchoscopy. Surgical resection is the treatment of choice and is usually curative.

TRACHEAL TUMOURS

Tracheal tumours present with breathlessness, wheeze, and stridor, and are commonly mistaken for asthma. The chest radiograph is often normal. Eighty percent of these tumours are malignant and grow very rapidly. Benign tumours present more insidiously. The diagnosis can be made using a flow volume loop that shows flattening of the expiratory curve, followed by bronchoscopy. Malignant tumours can be palliated with radiotherapy and benign tumours can be resected or debulked with laser treatment.

SUMMARY

- ❏ Lung cancer is the commonest fatal malignancy in men and women.
- ❏ Lung cancer is increasing in women as more women take up smoking.
- ❏ The majority of lung cancer patients present with advanced disease.
- ❏ Few lung cancer patients are offered curative surgery in the UK.
- ❏ All patients with advanced NSCLC and performance score < 2 should be offered platinum-based combination chemotherapy to treat symptoms and prolong survival.
- ❏ Smoking cessation and avoidance are the only evidence-based strategies to reduce the future incidence of lung cancer.
- ❏ Lung cancer screening with LDCT should only be offered in a clinical trial.

RECOMMENDED READING

British Thoracic Society Guidelines on diagnostic flexible bronchoscopy and on the management of those with lung cancer. www.brit-thoracic.org.uk

Diagnosis and management of lung cancer: ACCP evidence based guidelines. *Chest* **123**: 1 (suppl.) (2003).

Chapter 6 Chronic obstructive pulmonary disease

INTRODUCTION

The British Thoracic Society guidelines define chronic obstructive pulmonary disease (COPD) as 'a chronic slowly progressive disorder characterized by airways obstruction ($FEV_1 < 80\%$ predicted and FEV_1/VC ratio of $< 70\%$) which does not change markedly over several months'. In contrast to the airflow obstruction produced by asthma, airflow obstruction due to COPD is largely fixed.

COPD encompasses elements of the conditions chronic bronchitis and emphysema as well as some cases of chronic asthma, which have reached an irreversible stage (43). The terms chronic obstructive airways disease (COAD) and chronic obstructive lung disease (COLD) have been used in the past to denote the same condition but have now been superseded by the term COPD.

Chronic bronchitis is defined as a cough productive of sputum for 3 months in a year for at least 2 consecutive years, in the absence of other diseases recognized to cause sputum production.

Emphysema is defined, pathologically, as a condition characterized by irreversible dilatation of the air spaces distal to the terminal bronchiole with destruction of the alveolar walls, and without fibrosis.

Emphysema may be classified as:

❏ Panacinar: involves all the alveoli within the acinus equally (as happens with alpha-1 antitrypsin deficiency); commonly affects the lower lobes.
❏ Centriacinar: involves the alveoli near the respiratory bronchioles (as in smoking-induced emphysema); affects mainly the upper lobes.
❏ Paraseptal: involves the peripheral alveoli.

EPIDEMIOLOGY

COPD causes around 30,000 deaths a year in the UK. Prevalence increases with age, with 7.3% of males and 3.2% of females in the UK between 65 and 74 years of age suffering from the condition. One in eight medical admissions to hospital in the UK are due to an acute exacerbation of COPD, with the disease costing the NHS an estimated £500 million a year. Worldwide, COPD is the fourth leading cause of mortality; it is estimated that by the year 2020, COPD will be the 5th most common cause of disability among adults.

AETIOLOGY

CIGARETTE SMOKING

Smoking accounts for over 90% of all cases of COPD. While studies in the past have suggested that only

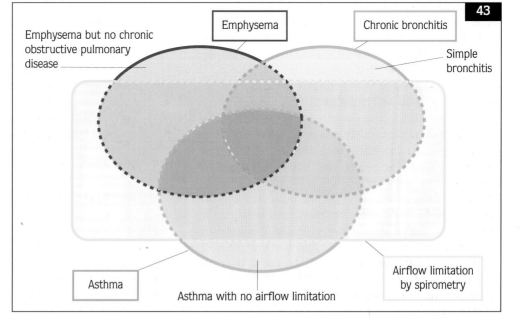

43 Airflow obstruction due to chronic bronchitis, asthma, and chronic obstructive pulmonary disease (COPD). The central shaded area denotes patients with airflow obstruction. Airflow obstruction as reflected by an FEV_1/VC ratio of $< 70\%$ is a must for the diagnosis of COPD. Note however that it is possible to suffer from chronic bronchitis and/or emphysema without spirometric evidence of COPD

43

Emphysema but no chronic obstructive pulmonary disease

Emphysema

Chronic bronchitis

Simple bronchitis

Asthma

Asthma with no airflow limitation

Airflow limitation by spirometry

around 15–25% of smokers develop COPD, more recent studies indicate that this figure might be nearer 50%, and even smokers without symptoms of COPD show a greater age-related decline in lung function than nonsmokers. Cigar and pipe smokers suffer a lower risk than cigarette smokers of developing COPD, but their risk of developing the disease remains higher than that of nonsmokers.

However, the fact that not all smokers develop the disease makes it likely that other genetic and/or environmental factors have a role to play in its development.

ALPHA-1 ANTITRYPSIN DEFICIENCY

Alpha-1 antitrypsin is an enzyme produced by the liver that maintains tissue integrity by preventing uncontrolled proteolytic destruction of the alveolar tissue (see below). An hereditary deficiency of the enzyme occurs in 1 in 5,000 live births in the UK and predisposes to destruction of the alveoli with resulting tendency to emphysema. The disease, which is inherited as an autosomal recessive condition, accounts for only 2% of all cases of emphysema and, even in those subjects who are homozygous for the condition, clinically significant emphysema usually occurs only when the subject is a cigarette smoker. Emphysema due to alpha-1 antitrypsin deficiency must be suspected in smokers who exhibit symptoms and signs of the disease at a relatively early age (under the age of 40) and those with a family history of emphysema.

OCCUPATIONAL FACTORS

Work in dusty environments, in particular the coal mining industry, is acknowledged as predisposing to the development of COPD. Other potential risk factors for developing COPD include pre-existing bronchial hyper-responsiveness, lower socio-economic status, and a poor nutritional status *in utero*.

PATHOLOGY AND PATHOGENESIS

The integrity of the alveolar tissue is dependent on a state of dynamic balance between tissue destruction and regeneration, mediated by a finely tuned system of proteolytic and anti-proteolytic enzymes (including alpha-1 antitrypsin). It is believed that COPD, in particular emphysema, develops in those subjects in whom toxin-induced inflammation has resulted in increased protease activity and a resultant imbalance between proteases and anti-proteases. It is unclear why it is only a small proportion of smokers who develop this protease-/anti-protease imbalance and it is likely that a number of other host and environmental factors may influence these processes (**44**).

CLINICAL FEATURES

PRESENTING SYMPTOMS

Breathlessness on exertion, cough, and sputum production are the main presenting features of COPD. However, significant COPD and lung dysfunction can exist in the absence of symptoms, particularly in sedentary individuals. Recurrent lower respiratory tract infections in smokers often draw them to the attention of the health services and, not uncommonly, a diagnosis of COPD is considered during such episodes.

Occasionally ankle swelling and features of cor pulmonale are the presenting symptoms.

PHYSICAL SIGNS OF COPD

❏ Changes in body habitus: 'pink puffer' (thin, tachypnoeic, and struggling to breathe – 'can't breathe') or 'blue bloater' (obese, cyanosed, drowsy – 'won't breathe').
❏ Ankle oedema and raised JVP in patients with cor pulmonale (see below).
❏ Hyperinflated ('barrel') chest (diminished distance from the top of the thyroid cartilage to the suprasternal notch; increased anteroposterior diameter of the thoracic cage).
❏ Symmetrically diminished lung expansion and air entry in both lung fields; wheeze.
❏ Increased forced expiratory time.

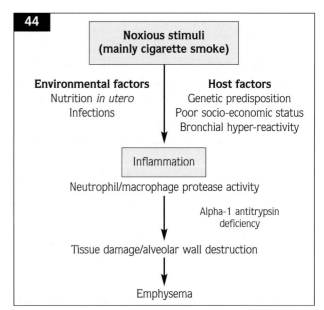

44 Factors involved in the aetiology and pathogenesis of chronic obstructive pulmonary disease

INVESTIGATIONS AND DIAGNOSIS

SPIROMETRY

Spirometry is central to the diagnosis of COPD (see Chapter 4). By definition COPD is characterized by an FEV_1/VC ratio of < 70% and an FEV_1 of < 80% predicted. In addition to helping define the presence of COPD, spirometry also enables the classification of COPD as mild, moderate or severe (**45**). FEV_1 as measured by spirometry is also a good prognostic indicator, with lower FEV_1 values being associated with poorer outcomes. In addition to airflow obstruction, emphysema is characterized by features of hyperinflation (increased residual volume [RV]) and reduced gas exchange (decreased TLCO and KCO). Reversibility testing involving performance of spirometry before and after a dose of inhaled bronchodilators is not routinely required to distinguish between COPD and asthma (**43**). However, an improvement of > 400 ml in FEV_1 following bronchodilator use in a patient with airflow

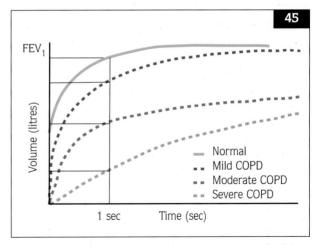

45 Spirometry showing a normal trace and features of mild, moderate, and severe chronic obstructive pulmonary disease (COPD)

obstruction may be indicative of asthma or an element of that condition.

CASE STUDIES

CASE STUDY 1

Ms HT is a 54-year-old woman with a smoking history of more than 35 pack-years. She sought her general practitioner's advice for a persistent headache following the loss of her job. She did not volunteer any symptoms referrable to her respiratory system but on specific questioning admitted to a 'smoker's cough' and breathlessness on moderate exertion. Opportunistic spirometry performed at the surgery showed airflow obstruction with no reversibility – an FEV_1 of 64% predicted with an FEV_1/VC ratio of 60%. A diagnosis of COPD was made and she was referred to the local smoking cessation clinic.

Interpretation:

❑ Opportunistic spirometry in smokers is useful in COPD case detection.

❑ Smoking cessation is the most effective treatment for COPD and should be actively pursued in all smokers with COPD.

OTHER INVESTIGATIONS IN COPD

Full blood count may show polycythaemia in some cases.

Chest radiograph is not required for the diagnosis of COPD but can help rule out other conditions that can cause breathlessness, including lung cancer and heart failure. In pure emphysema, the chest radiograph may show features of hyperinflation, with dark lung fields, flattened hemidiaphragms and a narrow cardiac shadow.

Pulse oximetry and arterial blood gas analysis: Long-term oxygen therapy (LTOT) may benefit some patients with moderate to severe COPD (see below), and assessment for this requires arterial blood gas analysis.

COPD patients with an oxygen saturation of < 92% on pulse oximetry should undergo blood gas analysis to assess suitability for LTOT (*Table 19*, page 55).

Significant oxygen desaturation may occur on exercise in some patients not on LTOT who have normal oxygen saturation at rest. Measurement of oxygen saturation on exercise, during a shuttle test, or 6-minute walking test may identify those patients for whom supplemental oxygen given during exertion may be of value. In these cases, testing is undertaken in a blinded manner with the patient exercising on air and oxygen, and a 10% improvement in symptoms or distance walked justifies the prescription of oxygen.

DIFFERENTIAL DIAGNOSIS

It can be difficult to distinguish asthma from COPD particularly in middle-aged smokers presenting with apparently episodic symptoms. *Table 16* lists features which can help distinguish between asthma and COPD (after the British Thoracic Society).

In a significant number of patients (as many as 20%), asthma can co-exist with COPD. Other conditions that need differentiation from COPD include heart failure (which can co-exist with COPD), bronchiectasis (see Chapter 11, page 119), and lung cancer (see Chapter 5, page 42).

MANAGEMENT

The aims of management are:
- ❑ To prevent progression of the disease.
- ❑ To reduce morbidity (relieve symptoms, improve exercise tolerance and health-related quality of life, including reduction of acute exacerbations and admissions to hospital).
- ❑ To reduce mortality.

SMOKING CESSATION

Smoking cessation is the single most effective treatment for COPD. Smokers who give up the habit by their early thirties not only avoid developing most of the smoking-related disease, but also prolong their life expectancy to levels comparable to those of nonsmokers. However after 20 years or more of smoking, absolute risks of death from COPD remain high even in those who give up the habit, although their risk is less than that of continuing smokers. The following have been shown to be effective in achieving smoking cessation:
- ❑ Advice from a health professional (doctor or nurse), however brief, results in 2% of smokers giving up the habit. Given that 70% of smokers attend primary care every year the potential benefit from this apparently low success rate is considerable.
- ❑ Nicotine replacement therapy (NRT): nicotine gums, sprays, transdermal patches, lozenges, and inhalers provide nicotine without tar and other chemicals. NRTs double 'quit rates' with no evidence to suggest that any one form of NRT is better than another.
- ❑ Bupropion is a dopaminergic and noradrenergic reuptake inhibitor that doubles cessation rates compared with placebo and when used with NRT. The alpha-2 noradrenergic agonist, clonidine, and the antidepressant, nortriptyline, have been used as second-line pharmacotherapeutic agents in aiding smoking cessation.

Table 17 describes the strategies used to help patients to cease smoking.

Table 16 Differential diagnosis of chronic obstructive pulmonary disease (COPD)

	COPD	Asthma
Heavy smoker or ex-smoker	Yes	Maybe
Was chesty as a child	Maybe	Often
Cough and sputum	For many years	Often recent
Breathlessness started	Gradually	Sudden attacks
Breathlessness varies	Little	A lot
Attacks of breathlessness at rest	Uncommon except at late stages	Common
Cough in the morning	Common	Uncommon
Cough at night	Uncommon	Common
FEV_1	Low	Low or normal
PEF	Maybe low	Low or normal
Daily variations in PEF	Little	'Morning dip' and day-to-day
Response to bronchodilators	Partial or none	Often significant
Eosinophilia	No	Usual
Effect of corticosteroids	Negligible	Improvement

PEF, peak expiratory flow

BRONCHODILATORS INCLUDING THEOPHYLLINES (SEE CHAPTER 15, PAGE 159)

Inhaled short-acting β-agonists (salbutamol and terbutaline), long-acting β-agonists (salmeterol and formoterol), anticholinergic agents (ipratropium, oxitropium, and tiotropium), and oral theophyllines have all been shown to improve symptoms of COPD. However none of the bronchodilators have been shown to alter the long-term history of the condition or affect mortality, although the new anticholinergic agent, tiotropium, may be an exception in this regard. There is no evidence to suggest that using one type of bronchodilator first is any better than another, but using a combination of a β-agonist and an anticholinergic agent is better than using either alone. It is also advisable to start with one agent and escalate the treatment rather than commence various agents all at once.

Inhaled corticosteroids have no significant effect on the rate of decline of lung function in COPD but may be useful in moderate to severe cases of COPD by preventing repeated acute exacerbations. Inhaled steroids are recommended for patients who have an FEV of < 50% predicted, and have had two or more exacerbations in the previous year.

Mucolytics such as N-acetylcysteine and carbocysteine are beneficial in reducing the symptoms of cough and sputum production in some patients.

PULMONARY REHABILITATION

A structured multi-disciplinary programme of exercise and education (including aspects of breathing control) has been shown to improve exercise capacity and quality of life, and to reduce hospitalization rates in patients with COPD (*Table 18*).

OXYGEN THERAPY

Studies performed over 30 years ago in the United Kingdom by the Medical Research Council (MRC) and in North America (the Nocturnal Oxygen Therapy Trial – NOTT) have shown that, in COPD patients with hypoxia and hypercapnia or features of cor pulmonale, the use of LTOT improved life expectancy. Based on these trials the Department of Health in the UK has drawn up some criteria for the use of LTOT (*Table 19*). LTOT is provided via an oxygen concentrator, which extracts oxygen from ambient air circumventing the need for cylinders of oxygen, or from a liquid oxygen supply. Oxygen is usually delivered via nasal cannulae at flow rates determined after specialist assessment. (NB: uncontrolled oxygen therapy can result in worsening of hypercapnia.) Those on LTOT may also

---

Table 17 Strategies to help the chronic obstructive pulmonary disease patient quit smoking (after the global initiative for chronic obstructive lung disease [GOLD] guidelines)

Ask:	Identify tobacco users at every visit
Advise:	To quit in a strong personalized manner
Assess:	Willingness to quit
Assist:	Provide access to counselling, nicotine replacement therapy, and pharmacotherapy
Arrange:	Follow up

Table 18 Elements of pulmonary rehabilitation programme and professionals involved

Elements of programme	Professional involved
Physical and exercise therapy, training of limb and respiratory muscles	Physiotherapist
Understanding the illness, strategies to stop smoking	Specialist nurse
Aids to daily living	Occupational therapist
Good use of medication	Specialist nurse and pharmacist
Dietary and nutritional advice	Dietitian
Relaxation techniques, psychotherapy	Clinical psychologist
Advice on oxygen therapy, assisted ventilation, lifestyle, and travel	Specialist nurse
Benefits advice and social support	Social worker

Table 19 Criteria for the use of long-term oxygen therapy

- ❏ Assessment to be made during clinical stability (not during an acute exacerbation)

- ❏ Smoking cessation and optimum bronchodilator therapy must be established

- ❏ DHSS criteria for long-term oxygen therapy: $FEV_1 < 1.5$ l; $VC < 2.0$ l; $PaO_2 < 7.3$ kPa; $PaCO_2 > 6$ kPa

- ❏ Oxygen should be used for at least 15 hours a day (preferably more) to confer survival benefit

require additional small cylinders of oxygen, or liquid oxygen supplies and oxygen conserving devices, so that they may breathe supplementary oxygen while undertaking exercise outside the home.

SURGERY

Lung volume reduction surgery (LVRS) to restore normal lung mechanics and reduce breathlessness, and lung transplantation are of value in a small number of patients with COPD. In emphysematous patients with large bullae, removal of the bulla (bullectomy) may improve lung function.

ACUTE EXACERBATIONS OF COPD

Most patient with moderate to severe COPD suffer at least two acute exacerbations of their condition each year, usually, but not exclusively, during the winter months. These exacerbations are caused by viral (influenza, parainfluenza and so on) or bacterial (*Haemophilus influenzae, Moraxella catarrhalis, Streptococcus pneumoniae,* and so on) infections and

can adversely affect the health of the COPD patient for a significant time afterwards. Management is with:
- ❑ Increased-dosage bronchodilators.
- ❑ Antibiotics (usually amoxicillin, erythromycin or a tetracycline).
- ❑ Oral steroids (usually prednisolone 30 mg), which reduce the duration of illness and enable earlier discharge if hospitalized.
- ❑ Controlled oxygen.
- ❑ In some cases with respiratory failure, assisted ventilation delivered either invasively, via an endotracheal tube (following sedation and paralysis), or noninvasively (via a nasal or face mask (Chapter 13, page 132).

SUMMARY OF MANAGEMENT OF COPD

There is a large number of interventions that can be used to the advantage of the patient with COPD (see below) (46). It is important that they are used at the appropriate stages of the illness, where they confer maximum benefit.

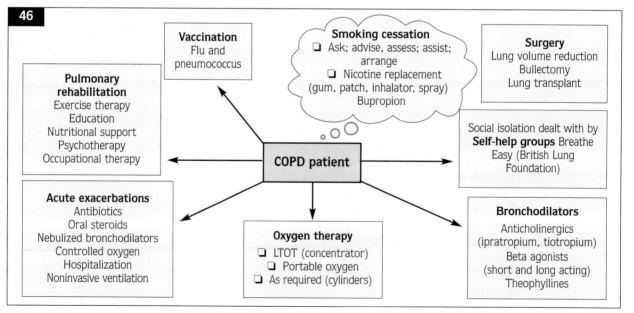

46 Management of chronic obstructive pulmonary disease (COPD)

COMPLICATIONS OF COPD

❏ Cor pulmonale: pulmonary hypertension and resultant failure of the right heart. Clinical signs: elevated jugular venous pressure, congestive hepatomegaly, and peripheral oedema.

❏ Respiratory failure: hypoxia ($PaO_2 < 8$ kPa) with or without hypercapnia ($PaCO_2 > 6$ kPa); acute exacerbations of COPD are a common cause of type II respiratory failure (hypoxia with hypercapnia).

❏ Weight loss and malnutrition occur in 10–25% of patients with COPD and are associated with poorer prognosis.

NATURAL HISTORY OF COPD

In the presence of continued smoking, FEV_1 decreases progressively at a rate of greater than 30 ml/year (average in a nonsmoker). Complications of COPD supervene, with progressive disability and death following (47).

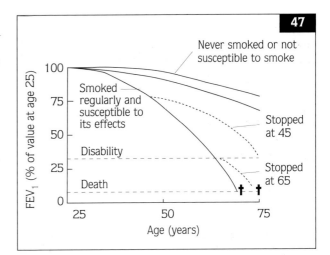

47 Natural history of COPD (after Fletcher & Peto. *BMJ* 1977;**i**:1645–1648).

SUMMARY

❏ COPD is a disease caused mainly by smoking. It is characterized by airflow obstruction which, in contrast to asthma, is mainly irreversible and progressive.

❏ The key to the diagnosis of COPD is spirometry, which demonstrates airflow obstruction (FEV_1/VC ratio of < 70% and/ or FEV_1 of < 80% predicted)

❏ Worldwide, COPD is the 4th most common cause of death and is predicted to become the 5th most common cause of disability by 2020.

❏ Smoking cessation is the most effective treatment for COPD and smoking cessation therapies (advice, NRT, and pharmacological treatments) are among the most cost-effective treatments in medicine.

❏ Pulmonary rehabilitation techniques, based on physical therapy and education, improve quality of life and reduce hospital admissions from the disease; bronchodilators improve symptoms.

❏ LTOT, given to set criteria, is the only treatment known to improve mortality in COPD.

❏ Acute exacerbations of COPD are a common cause of medical admissions to hospital; they are treated with increased-dosage bronchodilators, antibiotics, controlled oxygen therapy, oral steroids, and noninvasive ventilation.

RECOMMENDED READING

British Thoracic Society. British Thoracic Society guidelines on the management of COPD. *Thorax* 1997;**52** (Suppl 5):S1S–28.

Global Initiative for Chronic Obstructive Lung Disease (GOLD). *Global strategy for the diagnosis, management, and prevention of chronic obstructive pulmonary disease.* NHLBI/ WHO workshop report. NIH publication no. 2701A, March 2001.

Smoking cessation guidelines and their cost effectiveness. *Thorax* 1998;53(5).

NICE guidelines on COPD. Management of chronic obstructive pulmonary disease in adults in primary and secondary care. *Thorax* 2004;59(Suppl1):156.

Chapter 7 Asthma

INTRODUCTION

Asthma is notoriously difficult to define. It is a syndrome characterized by:

❏ Reversible airflow obstruction.
❏ Bronchial hyper-responsiveness.
❏ Airway inflammation.
❏ Asthma symptoms (wheeze, chest tightness, breathlessness, cough [productive/nonproductive]).

Airway calibre can vary either spontaneously over time or with treatment, inhaled bronchodilator or steroid. Bronchial hyper-responsiveness refers to increased bronchoconstrictor response (sensitivity and/or maximum response) to a variety of direct-acting stimuli, e.g. histamine, cholinergic agonists, leuko-trienes or prostaglandins, or indirect-acting agents, e.g. exercise, cold air hyperventilation, fog, metabisulphite, and so on. In practice, bronchial responsiveness is usually tested to histamine or methacholine in the laboratory, or to exercise in children. Its absence in a patient with untreated asthma should lead to reconsideration of the diagnosis.

Airway inflammation is considered to be pathogenetic in asthma, underlying the other abnormalities. Fibre-optic bronchoscopy, broncho-alveolar lavage, and bronchial biopsy have been used experimentally to assess airway inflammation in asthma. Induced or natural sputum eosinophil counts have been applied to the diagnosis and management of clinical asthma.

EPIDEMIOLOGY

Asthma is common, occurring in approximately 8% of adults and up to 20% of children in the UK. It is more common in boys up to puberty, when it becomes more common in girls. There is considerable variation in prevalence from country to country (5% in China, 39% in Tristan da Cunha) and race to race, and between urban and rural environments in developing countries but not in Western Europe. Adoption of a more affluent, Western lifestyle appears to lead to an increase in the prevalence of asthma. This effect occurs over 5 to 10 years, suggesting the importance of environmental factors. Possible environmental factors include maternal (and paternal) smoking, reduced rates of breast feeding, viral infections in early life, housing (ventilation), various allergens, particularly house dust mites, moulds, household pets (particularly cats), air

pollution (indoor and outdoor), diet, the 'hygiene hypothesis' (lack of childhood infectious exposure and altered T-cell function), immunizations, and so on.

Air pollution, (e.g. release of sulphur dioxide from power stations or traffic fumes) while a trigger, is not linked to the prevalence of asthma. The reunion of East and West Germany is the best experimental test of this; people of common genetic background with distinct established rates of atopy (eczema and rhinitis) and lower incidence of asthma in East Germany, despite very high levels of industrial pollution, assumed the four-fold higher West German levels of atopy and asthma, despite the lower pollution levels, within 5 years of reunion of the two countries.

Variations in the prevalence of asthma are also reflected in variations in death rates from asthma, though other factors, including medical care and accuracy of notification rates, may affect the statistics. To improve diagnostic accuracy asthma statistics are often compiled for patients between the ages of 5 and 34 years (since the diagnosis of asthma is uncertain in children below the age of 4–5, and COPD is very unlikely under the age of 35). Mortality rates have fluctuated widely within individual countries over the last 50 years. In England and Wales deaths due to asthma increased markedly in a 1960s 'epidemic' but then fell in the 1970s, rose again slightly in the early 1980s and fell during the 1990s, to about 1500 annually. The subsequent rise was mainly in older people and is likely to have reflected increased diagnosis of asthma; it was accompanied by an increase in hospital admissions in all age groups but particularly in children. This was not apparently due to a lower threshold for admission, as comparisons, if anything, showed increased severity. It has been pointed out that when prevalence increases markedly a very small change in overall severity may lead to dramatically increased severity in a sub-population with very severe or fatal asthma.

GENETIC FACTORS

Genetic factors are important but asthma genetics is complex. Asthma and particularly atopy clearly run in families. If both parents have asthma virtually 100% of their offspring will. Twin studies suggest that up to 60% of asthma susceptibility is inherited but as few as 19% of monozygotic twins are concordant for asthma. Many recent studies have linked different genes on chromosomes 5q, 7, 1, 11q,

12q, 16, 17, and 21q to various components of asthma, including clinical atopy, immunoglobulin-E (IgE) production, bronchial hyper-responsiveness, β_2 adrenoceptor function, and cytokine production.

AETIOLOGY

It is clear from the above that the cause(s) of asthma is/are unknown. Asthma is best regarded as a syndrome where the pathophysiology relates to airway inflammation.

Airway inflammation is characterized by T-helper cell (TH2) dysregulation and production of the interleukins IL-4, IL-5, and IL-13. In atopic asthma mast cells, by cross linking of high affinity immunoglobulin E (IgE) receptors, lead to the release of preformed mediators, e.g. histamine, tryptase, prostaglandins, and heparin, and synthesis of other mediators, including leukotrienes and platelet activating factors. In nonatopic (intrinsic) asthma there may be local IgE production in the bronchial mucosa. Eosinophils, which release tissue-damaging basic proteins, including major basic protein (MBP), eosinophil cationic protein (ECP), and eosinophil protein X (EPX), are thought to be key effector cells despite recent evidence that anti-IL-5 monoclonal antibody treatment was able to reduce greatly circulating eosinophils and reduce moderately airway eosinophil numbers without beneficial therapeutic effects in mild-to-moderate asthma.

Other cell types have been shown to be activated, e.g. alveolar macrophages and epithelial cells, which are also capable of releasing various cytokines. Polymorphonuclear neutrophil leucocytes are thought to be important, particularly in chronic, severe (steroid-dependent) asthma and about one third of acute exacerbations of asthma seem to be associated with increased airway neutrophils rather than eosinophils.

Characteristic structural changes are present even at an early stage in very mild disease, and these include patchy desquamated epithelium and thickening of the reticular collagen layer of the basement membrane. Goblet cell hyperplasia, increased numbers of mucus glands, new vessel formation, and hypertrophy and hyperplasia of airway smooth muscle are features of persistent asthma. Functional abnormalities include increased airway permeability, plasma exudation, enhanced parasympathetic and inhibitory nonadrenergic nervous pathways, and airway hyper-responsiveness.

CLINICAL FEATURES

HISTORY

The history is of particular importance in asthma, focusing on documenting the symptoms, their severity, triggering factors, past history of exacerbations, childhood and family history, and possible causes, e.g. allergies and occupational exposures.

Asthma symptoms include wheeze, cough (which may be an isolated symptom), sputum production, breathlessness, and chest tightness. Asthma symptoms typically vary in time and are intermittent. They are characteristically worse at night or in the early hours of the morning (0200–0400 hours). In taking a history these symptoms are enquired about with emphasis on their variability. This may be more difficult to obtain in older patients with more chronic asthma, in whom symptoms may be attributed to concomitant COPD. A childhood history of 'bronchitis' or inability to do school sports may be suggestive. A background of atopy, i.e. hay fever or eczema, or a positive family history is helpful (see *Table 16*, page 54, for differentiating asthma from COPD). In addition, potential triggers must be considered (*Table 20*).

Exposure to trigger factors can precipitate symptoms, particularly wheeze, chest tightness, and shortness of breath. Triggers include viral infections, common allergens (including seasonal effects – spring for pollens, autumn for moulds), exercise (particularly in younger adults or children), irritants, pollution (indoor or outdoor), food (particularly fruit, nuts, and shellfish), fizzy drinks, cold drinks, wine, beers, and food preservatives and colourings (e.g. metabisulphite, tartrazine, and monosodium glutamate). Hormonal factors, in terms of pregnancy or premenstrual worsening should be enquired about. Every patient should be asked about their response to nonsteroidal anti-inflammatory drugs (NSAIDs) and

---

Table 20 Asthma triggers

- ❏ Upper respiratory tract infections
- ❏ Exercise, particularly in cold weather
- ❏ Allergens – commonly dust, pollen, cats, and dogs
- ❏ Nonsteroidal anti-inflammatory drugs
- ❏ β-receptor blockers (including eye drops for glaucoma)
- ❏ Occupational factors
- ❏ Food, fizzy drinks, orange flavouring, ghee, peanuts
- ❏ Irritants, e.g. perfume, pollution, cigarette smoke, car fumes
- ❏ Changes in the weather, e.g. thunderstorms
- ❏ Before periods in menstruating women
- ❏ Stress

also occupational (see below) or environmental exposures. Common complicating coexisting conditions include smoking, rhinosinusitis, and gastro-oesophageal reflux.

Asthma is also characterized by exacerbations or attacks. There are no agreed precise definitions, but exacerbations refer to increased symptoms and increased airway narrowing, lasting a matter of days and requiring an increase in therapy.

CLINICAL EXAMINATION

Physical examination is of little help in the diagnosis of intermittent asthma, as it is usually normal. When bronchial obstruction is present there may be expiratory wheeze, which is caused by turbulent airflow in airways that are not completely constricted. Typically it is polyphonic as it arises from multiple, different-sized airways. A single fixed wheeze should raise the possibility of another cause of airway obstruction, for example tumour or foreign body. Other auscultatory findings are not features of asthma and require explanation. Chest deformity in adults arising from chronic severe airflow obstruction in childhood is now rare. Features of acute severe asthma are dealt with later.

INVESTIGATIONS AND DIAGNOSIS

Investigations may be simple. Demonstration of airflow obstruction which varies over time or with treatment is a prerequisite. This may involve measuring peak expiratory flow (PEF) before and after an inhaled β_2 agonist (e.g. two puffs [200 µg] of salbutamol) to demonstrate bronchodilator reversibility. Spirometry may be more sensitive. Home monitoring of PEF, may be diagnostic. The patient should record the best of three measurements first thing on waking, and again in the afternoon or evening for comparison. The best of three measurements is also recorded at the time of symptoms (e.g. at night), and 5 minutes after an inhaled β_2 agonist. Spirometry is also useful for showing the variability and pattern of airflow obstruction and response to therapy and in teaching patients about self-management.

A chest radiograph is indicated in newly presenting adult asthma to exclude alternative diagnoses, e.g. a tumour in a smoker, or to document complications (*Tables 21* and *22*).

Table 21 Important differential diagnoses in asthma

- ❏ Chronic obstructive pulmonary disease (COPD)
- ❏ Viral wheeze, particularly in young children
- ❏ Hyperventilation
- ❏ Bronchiectasis
- ❏ Main airway obstruction, e.g. bronchial carcinoma, bronchial adenoma, or foreign body (especially in a child)
- ❏ Heart failure
- ❏ Laryngeal dysfunction
- ❏ Upper airway obstruction
- ❏ Pulmonary embolism
- ❏ Pneumothorax
- ❏ Eosinophilic bronchitis
- ❏ Primary pulmonary hypertension

Table 22 Complications of asthma

Acute
- ❏ Acute exacerbation(s)
- ❏ Mucus plugging
    atelectasis or collapse
- ❏ Pneumothorax
    surgical emphysema
    mediastinal emphysema
- ❏ Cough trauma
    e.g. rib fracture (osteoporosis)
    subconjunctival haemorrhage
- ❏ Acute respiratory failure
- ❏ Central nervous system
    confusion, coma, cerebral
        vascular accident

- ❏ Iatrogenic
    drugs
        psychosis
        gastrointestinal bleeding
    mechanical ventilation
        adverse effects
        infection
- ❏ ITU syndromes
    neuromuscular
- ❏ Psychosocial
- ❏ Death

Chronic
- ❏ Chronic progressive airflow
    obstruction
        increased FEV_1 decline
        emphysema on CT scan
        bronchiectasis

- ❏ Chronic cough
    hernias
    vaginal prolapse
- ❏ Iatrogenic
    corticosteroid side-effects
    immunosuppression
- ❏ Disability
    immobility
    de-conditioning
    obesity
- ❏ Psychosocial
    anxiety/depression
    isolation
    unemployment
- ❏ Gastro-oesophageal reflux
- ❏ Ischaemic heart disease
- ❏ Cor pulmonale (very rare)
- ❏ Premature death

Sensitivity to common allergens is usually examined by prick skin tests. Specific IgE is measured by the radioallergosorbent test (RAST). These have advantages and disadvantages but are expensive and should not be used routinely. Atopy is present in around 40% of the UK population. A full blood count is useful, as discovery of a raised eosinophil count may indicate a need for other tests (*Table 23*).

Examination of a satisfactory sputum sample, produced spontaneously or induced by inhalation of hypertonic saline (after β_2 agonist pre-treatment because saline may induce bronchoconstriction) may reveal direct evidence of eosinophilic airway inflammation but it is not a standard test.

When airway function is normal bronchial challenge may be useful but it has limited sensitivity and specificity (see Chapter 15, page 159). Exercise testing is particularly useful in children.

A corticosteroid trial (e.g. 2 weeks of prednisolone 30–40 mg daily or 6 weeks of a high-dose inhaled steroid) may uncover hidden reversibility of airflow obstruction which persists after use of a β_2 agonist alone.

It is essential to confirm the diagnosis of asthma objectively or management may be pursued with inappropriate escalation of therapy. The diagnosis depends on the demonstration of variable airflow obstruction. Airflow is measured by FEV_1 or PEF and then re-measured 5–15 minutes after inhalation of a standard dose of a β_2 agonist (e.g. salbutamol 200 µg from an inhaler and chamber device, or 2.5 mg by nebulizer or terbutaline 1 mg by turbohaler). Provided the measurements are technically reliable, an increase in FEV_1 of > 15% (and > 200 ml) or PEF of > 20% can be considered diagnostic. Alternatively, a variation of 20% in amplitude % best PEF (with a minimum change of 60 l/minute) may be diagnostic. PEF is recorded at home, first thing in the morning and later in the day, on 3 or more days per week over 2 weeks. Percentage best PEF is calculated as follows:

$$\frac{(\text{highest PEF} - \text{lowest PEF}) \times 100}{\text{highest PEF}}$$

If airflow is initially within the normal range, variability can be established by bronchial challenge to establish hyper-responsiveness compared to normal individuals. In the laboratory histamine, methacholine, or exercise, are the most commonly used challenges. Strictly, asthma is diagnosed by the presence of compatible symptoms and establishing hyper-responsiveness. Similarly, the conjunction of compatible symptoms and induced or spontaneous sputum eosinophilia (> 3%), together with response to asthma therapy, constitutes an operational diagnostic algorithm. Because of asthma's variable nature, trial of therapy is perfectly reasonable. If symptoms persist, objective testing to establish or exclude the diagnosis is mandatory.

DIFFERENTIAL DIAGNOSIS

Important differential diagnoses (*Table 21*) to consider include: COPD, viral wheeze (particularly in young children), upper airway obstruction, bronchiectasis, main airway obstruction (e.g. bronchial carcinoma in a smoker), benign tumour (e.g. adenoma), a foreign body or a compressive lesion. Other common conditions to consider include heart failure (often with wheeze and nocturnal exaggeration) and pulmonary embolism (there may

---

Table 23 Eosinophilia in asthma

Eosinophil count ($\times 10^9$/l)	Associated condition
0.0–0.4	Normal
0.5–0.8	Consistent with atopy
> 1.5	Pulmonary eosinophilia or vasculitis (?)
> 5–20	Hypereosinophilia Haemopoietic malignancy (?)

Further investigations	
Chest radiograph	To look for infiltrates allergic bronchopulmonary aspergillosis (?)
Total IgE	Usually elevated in allergy if markedly elevated parasites (?)
Serology for	*Filariasis* *Strongyloides* *Schistosoma*
Fresh stool examinations	For eggs and larvae
Skin tests	To look for specific allergies
RAST	For allergy (particularly *Aspergillus*)
CRP	Very elevated in active vasculitis
ANCA	Churg–Strauss syndrome

ANCA, antineutrophil anticytoplasmic antibodies; CRP, C reactive protein; IgE, immunoglobulin E; RAST, radioallergosorbent test

be stuttering in milder, chronic cases). Rarer but important conditions include eosinophilic bronchitis (cough and eosinophilic sputum but no variability of airflow obstruction or hyper-responsiveness) and primary pulmonary hypertension (unexplained breathlessness in a young woman which may apparently remit).

Because asthma is so common it often coexists with other conditions, particularly COPD and hyperventilation (a consistent feature of acute asthma). Laryngeal dysfunction (glottic wheezing) is a condition which coexists with asthma. It is not uncommon, particularly in women associated with the health care professions. This serves to emphasize the importance of objectively establishing the diagnosis.

MANAGEMENT OF CHRONIC ASTHMA

The aims of asthma management can be summarized as:

❑ Absence (or minimization) of symptoms.
❑ Normalization (or maximization) of lung function.
❑ Absence (or minimization) of exacerbations.
❑ No (or minimal) limitations to lifestyle.
❑ Minimization of drug dosages.
❑ Absence (or minimization) of drug side-effects.

There is increasing interest in non-pharmacological management, which includes avoidance of causes, such as allergens or occupational inducers, triggers, and nondrug treatments.

COMPLEMENTARY THERAPY

There is much current interest in the use of complementary (alternative) therapy and many people with asthma have tried one or more approaches. Unfortunately, there is a dearth of high-quality clinical trial evidence. Small benefits have been shown in some studies for acupuncture, Chinese herbal medicine, and hypnosis, but no definite clinical role has been established. Breathing exercises are popular with patients. Yoga and Buteyko techniques aim to reduce hyperventilation by reducing respiratory rate. A number of studies have shown some benefit; yoga (pranayama) reduced airway responsiveness and Buteyko techniques have reduced β_2 agonist use and exacerbations, and improved symptoms, without altering lung function. Physical training does not increase lung function but improves cardiopulmonary function, oxygen consumption, maximum heart rate, and work capacity.

Air ionizers have not proved beneficial. Homoeopathy and hypnosis remain of unproven value, though benefits have been claimed. Chiropractice and massage therapy have no proven place in management. Speleotherapy (exposure to cave environments) cannot yet be recommended.

DIET

High salt intake is correlated with asthma severity and bronchial responsiveness. In a controlled trial adding salt to a low-salt diet caused minor physiological deterioration. Low magnesium and selenium levels have been associated with asthma but only magnesium supplementation produced minor benefit. Fish oil (omega n-3 fatty acids) supplementation has proved ineffective. Weight reduction in obese patients was beneficial in a small, randomized parallel group study in severe asthma.

ALLERGEN AVOIDANCE

Primary prophylaxis refers to an intervention aimed at preventing the development of a condition. In the case of asthma this relates to the prevention of allergic sensitization in early life by reducing exposure to allergens. The results of a study of the avoidance of house dust mites in early pregnancy to reduce asthma development in infancy are awaited.

Exposure to allergens is associated with increased severity of existing asthma, increased treatment requirements, hospital attendance, and respiratory arrest. House dust mite allergen control is difficult, but can be achieved with a combination of measures, including mattress and pillow covers, removal of carpets and soft toys, high temperature washing of bed linen, dehumidification, special vacuuming, and acaricides on soft furnishings. However, clinical benefit is unproven and unlikely to be cost-effective.

Removal of pets is usually advised, although evidence from controlled trials is lacking and, in theory, high levels of exposure to cats may induce immunological tolerance.

IMMUNOTHERAPY

Allergen-specific immunotherapy (desensitization) with increasing doses of allergens given subcutaneously is rarely used in the UK compared with Europe and the US. Its attraction is modification of the underlying immunopathology and the natural history of the disease. It shows consistent small benefits in reducing symptoms and use of medication in controlled trials. However, there are no good comparisons with conventional pharmacotherapy. The benefits of immunotherapy in treatment-resistant allergic rhinitis are much greater than in asthma, which is rarely related to a single allergen, though isolated sensitivity (e.g. to cats) may be improved.

Adverse effects, which can prove fatal, range from anaphylaxis occurring in minutes, to skin reactions, rhinitis or delayed-onset asthma. Cost–benefit analyses are not available.

PHARMACOLOGICAL THERAPY

A step-wise approach to treatment has long been used and is advocated by national and international guidelines. Patients are started at treatment appropriate to their level of severity. In fact, asthma severity is difficult to define or measure as it has to take into account the amount of treatment and the degree of control achieved. The aim is for the early abolition of symptoms and normalization of lung function, stepping down treatment when good control has been achieved, and stepping up treatment as necessary. The latest British asthma guideline summarizes treatment of asthma in all age groups very adequately and is evidence based. The five steps and treatment recommendations are illustrated in figure **48**. In brief:

Step 1 represents mild intermittent asthma, for which inhaled short-acting β_2 agonists (e.g. salbutamol or terbutaline) are the preferred bronchodilators over anticholinergics, theophylline, oral β_2 agonists, and anti-leukotrienes. Inhaled β_2 agonists or 'relievers' are prescribed as required. Overuse (more than two canisters per month or 10–12 puffs daily) indicates poorly controlled asthma, though the consensus is that β_2 agonists are not harmful given regularly, as often as four times daily.

Step 2 requires the introduction of regular 'preventer' therapy. Inhaled corticosteroids are preferred as the most effective option. The threshold for their introduction has not been established, but they are indicated for patients requiring inhaled β_2 agonists more than twice daily, with nocturnal symptoms, after a recent exacerbation, with sub-optimal lung function.

Treatment is usually started at beclometasone (BDP) equivalent 200 µg twice daily. The dose can be given as a single dose, preferably at night, once good control is achieved. Some patients have concerns about the safety of inhaled steroids, largely as a reflection of the well known side-effects of oral steroid therapy. These fears are unfounded below a dose of 800 µg daily in adults (400 µg daily in children).

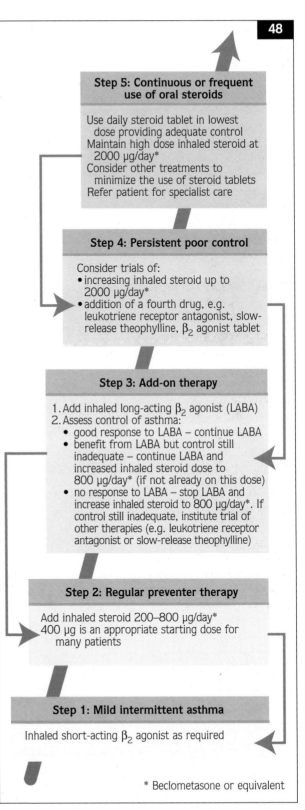

48 Summary of stepwise management of asthma in adults

Local side-effects of inhaled steroids may include:
- Sore throat.
- Dysphonia (hoarseness) due to reversible larnygeal muscle dysfunction.
- Oropharyngeal candidiasis (thrush).

These can usually be resolved by altering the delivery device or changing to a different inhaled steroid and encouraging mouth rinsing to remove locally deposited drug.

Suppression of plasma cortisol is a pharmacological effect of inhaled steroids. This demonstrates a systemic action of the inhaled drugs, indicating systemic absorption. The degree varies very considerably between different individuals, between patients and normal subjects, and for different inhaled steroids and delivery devices. It is of uncertain clinical significance, though adrenal insufficiency has been reported in a small number of children presenting with hypoglycaemia who had been treated with doses in excess of the licensed indication. Other potential side-effects are shown in *Table 24*.

Table 24 Potential side-effects of inhaled corticosteroids

Local inhaled steroid side-effects
- Sore throat
- Dysphonia
- Candidiasis

Systemic inhaled steroid side-effects
- Bruising
- Osteoporosis
- Growth suppression
- Cortisol suppression
- Glaucoma
- Dental problems
- 'Addiction'
- Steroid phobia
- Psychosis

Oral steroid side-effects
- Weight gain
- Diabetes
- Infection/immunosuppression
- Cataracts
- Hirsutism
- Hypertension
- Oedema

Other preventer therapies include:
- **Cromones,** such as sodium cromoglycate and nedocromil sodium.
- **Leukotriene receptor antagonists (LTRAs),** e.g. zafirlukast and montelukast.
- **Theophyllines,** including a variety of slow-release preparations.
- **Inhaled long-acting β2 agonists,** salmeterol and formoterol.
- **Antihistamines** – conventional, selective non-sedating, and ketotifen; all of which are ineffective.

Step 3 relates to 'add on' therapy, which should only be considered once inhaler technique and compliance with existing therapy have been checked. A variety of studies have shown that addition of a long-acting β_2 agonist is superior to doubling (or more than doubling) the dose of inhaled steroid across a range of asthma severities, different starting doses, and compounds. Improvements in lung function, symptoms, and quality of life, and reductions in exacerbations have been shown. A trial of an inhaled long-acting β_2 agonist is recommended at inhaled steroid doses between 200 and 800 µg daily. This is the first choice option for adults and children aged 5–12 years.

In patients who have been shown to benefit from addition of an inhaled long-acting β_2 agonist to an inhaled steroid, a combination of the two in a single inhaler (Seretide: salmeterol/fluticasone, Symbicort: formoterol/budesonide) is logical, simpler, popular with patients, cost-saving, and may improve compliance.

The addition of LTRAs and theophyllines to inhaled steroids has been shown to be equivalent to doubling the dose of inhaled steroid. Both improve lung function and symptoms while LTRAs have been shown to reduce exacerbations. Theophylline and oral long-acting β_2 agonists (slow-release salbutamol or terbutaline or the pro-drug bambuterol) are associated with more side-effects.

Step 4 is addition of a fourth drug. A small number of patients have asthma uncontrolled by an inhaled steroid 800 µg/day and an inhaled long-acting β_2 agonist. There are few controlled trials, but options include increasing the dose of inhaled steroids, adding an LTRA, a theophylline, or an oral long-acting β_2 agonist. If benefit cannot be shown from any addition then the drug should be stopped. Patients at this step should be considered for referral to a specialist.

Stepping down inhaled steroids

Little evidence is available regarding the timing of 'stepping down' the dose of inhaled steroids once asthma is controlled. Reducing the dose by about 25–50% at intervals of 3 months has been recommended without much evidence. There is evidence that without active monitoring of the stepping down of therapy, some patients are over-treated.

Stepping up

Most studies of self-management which have involved a patient receiving a written personal asthma action plan, have included as one action doubling the dose of inhaled steroid at the first sign of deterioration. These studies have shown improved outcomes. However, doubling the dose of inhaled steroid as the sole intervention does not prevent asthma worsening. This paradox is unexplained, but most guidelines recommend increasing the dose of an inhaled steroid at the first sign of deterioration. More than doubling the dose may be necessary to prevent the development of, or to treat, an exacerbation. One study showed budesonide 100 µg twice daily to be as effective as 400 µg twice daily over a 6-month period, if the dose of budesonide was increased five-fold for 2 weeks at the first sign of an asthma exacerbation. This clearly allows a considerable reduction in steroid intake long-term for the majority of patients. A five-fold increase in dose cannot be recommended for patients taking higher initial doses. However, in one study of general practice patients taking an initial, average inhaled steroid dose of 800 µg BDP, adding fluticasone 2,000 µg daily via spacer was as effective in treating an exacerbation as adding prednisolone 40 mg daily, reducing over 16 days.

Currently, the dose of inhaled steroid is adjusted according to the degree of asthma control gauged according to traditional measures – level of symptoms, use of β_2 agonist 'reliever', peak flow (with or without FEV_1), and recent history of exacerbations. The possibility of incorporating other measures of the inflammatory process has recently been addressed. In the future it is possible that more specific measurements, e.g. of airway inflammation directly (induced sputum) or surrogates (methacholine responsiveness or exhaled nitric oxide), may be used.

Step 5 relates to continuous or frequent use of oral steroids (prednisolone). Adverse effects are detailed in *Table 24*.

Common concomitant conditions, such as rhinosinusitis (present in 100% of steroid-dependent asthmatics), eczema, and gastro-oesophageal reflux (often silent), may also require treatment, though asthma control is usually unaffected.

INHALER DEVICES

Drug administration by the inhaled route provides a degree of selectivity with a greater effect, more rapidly, at a lower dose and hence fewer side-effects; e.g. salbutamol 200 µg by inhalation is more effective than salbutamol 4 mg (4,000 µg) orally. A large variety of different types of inhaler device exists to deliver drugs directly to the site of action in the airways. No single device is ideal for every patient. The pressurized metered dose inhaler (pMDI) remains the cheapest and most widely used, though many patients are unable to use it satisfactorily. It is essential that inhaler technique is checked at every opportunity and, if sub-optimal, further instruction or a change of device is necessary. A large volume spacer removes the need for co-ordination of activation of the pMDI and inspiration, increases pulmonary drug deposition, reduces oropharyngeal impaction (and local side-effects of inhaled steroids), and may reduce systemic side-effects (in the case of beclometasone). However, the large volume spacer devices (Volumatic, Nebuhaler) are specific to particular pharmaceutical company products and their size makes them unpopular with patients. Spacers should be washed in detergent and air dried monthly and replaced every 6–12 months. Some pMDIs come with integral spacers. Special aids, e.g. the Haleraid, enable the elderly or patients with arthritis to use a pMDI.

pMDIs are complex devices comprising metering chambers, valves, mixtures of propellants, and various stabilizing agents in addition to the drug itself. Traditional chlorofluorocarbon (CFC) propellants are being replaced by CFC-free hydroxyfluororalkane (HFA) pMDIs, in accordance with the Montreal convention to limit free radical damage to the ozone layer. These behave slightly differently from the older devices, with slower speed of discharge, altered taste, and different particle size.

For patients unable or unwilling to use pMDIs there is a wide choice of breath-actuated and dry powder devices. Specialist asthma nurses have a major role in training in the use of inhaler devices. This is essential, as patient preference for a particular device may often dictate the choice of drug within a pharmacological class.

PATIENT EDUCATION AND SELF-MANAGEMENT

Patient education involves a partnership between the patient and health care professional to enable guided self-management. This means empowering patients to control their own condition. Individualized advice needs to be given within the context of wider asthma education, culminating in a written personal action plan (**49**). Information must be tailored to the individual's needs respecting their right to determine how much control over their own condition they wish to take. Personal expectations should be elicited. Patients must be taught how to use their medication and be given advice about how to avoid triggers, recognize worsening asthma, and monitor their condition. Goals for treatment should be negotiated. In the light of the patient's wishes a written personal asthma action plan is devised. For some patients this might simply mean written reinforcement of clear advice to seek medical attention if they notice awakening, owing to asthma, at night. For others, increased use of their reliever should trigger medical attendance. For others, a more detailed written asthma action plan, incorporating PEF thresholds, for increase or decrease of inhaled steroid therapy, and initiation of

---

49

ZONE 1
Your asthma is under control if
- ❏ it does not disturb your sleep
- ❏ it does not restrict your usual activities and
- ❏ your peak flow reading is above _____

ACTION
Continue your normal medicines
Your preventer is

_____

You should normally take
___ puffs/doses
___ times every day (using a spacer), even when you are
feeling well
Your reliever is

_____

You should normally only take it when you are short of breath, coughing or wheezing, or before exercise
Your other medicines are

_____

_____

ZONE 2
Your doctor or nurse may decide not to use this zone
Your asthma is getting worse if
- ❏ you are needing to use your

_____

(reliever inhaler) more than usual
- ❏ you are waking at night with asthma symptoms, and
- ❏ your peak flow reading has fallen to
between _____ and _____

ACTION
Increase your normal medicines
- ❏ Increase your

_____

(preventer inhaler) to

_____

- ❏ Continue to take your

_____

(reliever inhaler) to relieve your asthma symptoms

ZONE 3
Your asthma is severe if
- ❏ you are getting increasingly breathless
- ❏ you are needing to use your

_____

(reliever inhaler) every
___ hours or more often, and
- ❏ your peak flow readings have fallen to
between _____ and _____

ACTION
Start a course of steroid tablets
- ❏ Take
___ prednisolone (steroid) tablets
(strength ____ mg each) and then

_____

_____

- ❏ Discuss with your doctor how and when to stop taking the tablets
- ❏ Continue to take your

_____

(reliever and preventer inhalers) as prescribed

ZONE 4
It is a medical emergency if
- ❏ your symptoms get worse, and
- ❏ your peak flow readings have fallen to below

_____

Do not be afraid of causing a fuss.
Your doctor will want to see you urgently.

ACTION
Get help immediately
- ❏ Telephone your doctor straightaway on

_____

or call an ambulance
- ❏ Take
____ prednisolone (steroid) tablets
(strength ____ mg each) immediately
- ❏ Continue to take your

_____

(reliever inhaler) as needed, or every five to ten minutes until the ambulance arrives

49 Example of an individual patient action plan

a course of oral steroids, or urgent presentation for medical attention, may be more appropriate.

The evidence in favour of self-management is overwhelming, particularly in more severe asthma. A large number of randomized controlled trials have shown that hospitalizations, emergency room visits, unscheduled visits to the doctor, and days off work or school can be reduced.

COMPLICATIONS

Asthma complications are shown in *Table 22*, page 60.

OSTEOPOROSIS SCREENING AND TREATMENT

All patients need general advice to prevent osteoporosis, though the risk is much greater in patients taking regular oral steroids or requiring frequent courses. Family history, smoking history, exercise (or its absence), alcohol intake, and adequate diet are important factors. It is important to obtain a baseline bone density by dual energy X-ray photon absorption (DEXA) scan to establish the diagnosis and severity – or refute it – and to plan treatment accordingly.

Increased risk of hip and spine fracture is seen on continuous daily doses of prednisolone as low as 7.5 mg. Loss of bone mineral density (BMD) is maximal in the first few weeks of oral steroid therapy. Steroids increase the risk of fracture above and beyond the BMD.

Management is summarized in figure 50. General measures include limiting the dose of oral prednisolone to the minimum, ensuring adherence

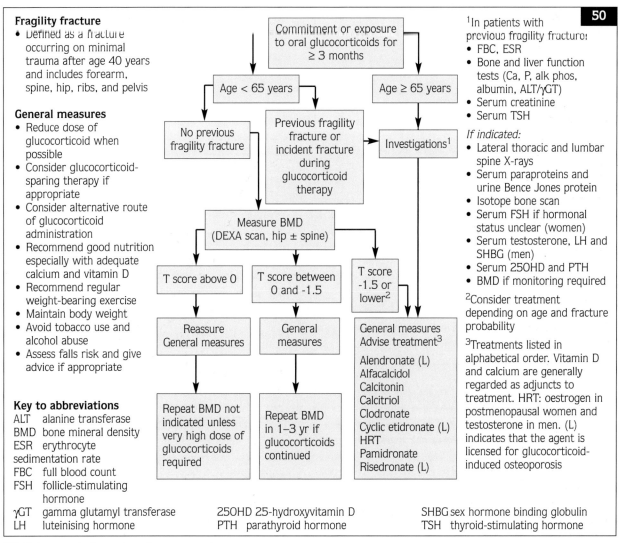

50

Fragility fracture
- Defined as a fracture occurring on minimal trauma after age 40 years and includes forearm, spine, hip, ribs, and pelvis

General measures
- Reduce dose of glucocorticoid when possible
- Consider glucocorticoid-sparing therapy if appropriate
- Consider alternative route of glucocorticoid administration
- Recommend good nutrition especially with adequate calcium and vitamin D
- Recommend regular weight-bearing exercise
- Maintain body weight
- Avoid tobacco use and alcohol abuse
- Assess falls risk and give advice if appropriate

Key to abbreviations
ALT alanine transferase
BMD bone mineral density
ESR erythrocyte sedimentation rate
FBC full blood count
FSH follicle-stimulating hormone
γGT gamma glutamyl transferase
LH luteinising hormone

Commitment or exposure to oral glucocorticoids for ≥ 3 months

Age < 65 years → No previous fragility fracture / Previous fragility fracture or incident fracture during glucocorticoid therapy

Age ≥ 65 years → Investigations[1]

Measure BMD (DEXA scan, hip ± spine)

T score above 0 → Reassure General measures → Repeat BMD not indicated unless very high dose of glucocorticoids required

T score between 0 and -1.5 → General measures → Repeat BMD in 1–3 yr if glucocorticoids continued

T score -1.5 or lower[2] → General measures Advise treatment[3]
Alendronate (L)
Alfacalcidol
Calcitonin
Calcitriol
Clodronate
Cyclic etidronate (L)
HRT
Pamidronate
Risedronate (L)

[1]In patients with previous fragility fracture:
- FBC, ESR
- Bone and liver function tests (Ca, P, alk phos, albumin, ALT/γGT)
- Serum creatinine
- Serum TSH

If indicated:
- Lateral thoracic and lumbar spine X-rays
- Serum paraproteins and urine Bence Jones protein
- Isotope bone scan
- Serum FSH if hormonal status unclear (women)
- Serum testosterone, LH and SHBG (men)
- Serum 25OHD and PTH
- BMD if monitoring required

[2]Consider treatment depending on age and fracture probability

[3]Treatments listed in alphabetical order. Vitamin D and calcium are generally regarded as adjuncts to treatment. HRT: oestrogen in postmenopausal women and testosterone in men. (L) indicates that the agent is licensed for glucocorticoid-induced osteoporosis

25OHD 25-hydroxyvitamin D
PTH parathyroid hormone

SHBG sex hormone binding globulin
TSH thyroid-stimulating hormone

50 Osteoporosis diagnosis and management

with high-dose inhaled steroids, considering steroid-sparing drugs, advice regarding good nutrition, particularly adequate calcium and vitamin D, weight-bearing exercise, maintaining body weight, stopping smoking, avoiding excess alcohol, and advice regarding falls if the risk is assessed as high. Steroid-induced bone loss has been shown to be prevented or reduced by treatment with calcium and vitamin D, alendronate, cyclic etidronate, risedronate, pamidronate, hormone replacement therapy, alpha-calcidol, calcitonin, and a number of other agents.

NATURAL HISTORY AND PROGNOSIS

The natural history of asthma is incompletely known as there are few good cohort studies. Most chronic asthma begins before the age of 10 years. Approximately 50% of children go into remission but the prognosis is worse the earlier the age of onset, if they are atopic or have more severe asthma, and the longer the follow up. In adults decline in FEV_1 is accelerated with smoking, and increased bronchial hyper-responsiveness.

SPECIFIC ASTHMA PROBLEMS

EXERCISE-INDUCED ASTHMA

Exercise-induced asthma (EIA) is an asthma syndrome, rather than a specific condition, which occurs more commonly in younger fitter adults or children. Typically EIA occurs after heavy exercise in the first 3–5 minutes after a 6-minute running test in the laboratory. The degree of bronchoconstriction induced depends on the type of exercise, the intensity and duration of exercise, the overall ventilation achieved, and the temperature and humidity of the inspired air, as well as underlying asthma severity.

The mechanism is incompletely understood but involves heat and water loss from the airway; EIA is closely reproduced by hyperventilation with dry air at subfreezing temperatures. The involvement of mast cell mediators is suggested by the inhibitory effects of specific antagonists of histamine and leukotrienes, and also by the phenomenon of the refractory period, when repetition of the same stimulus within a short time will not reproduce the same degree of bronchoconstriction.

The treatment of EIA follows the usual principles of asthma management. The dose of inhaled steroid may need increasing since EIA usually reflects poor control of the underlying condition. Exceptions to this occur when EIA may be the only expression of the disease, e.g. in elite athletes. EIA is prevented chronically by inhaled steroids, and acutely by inhaled short-acting β_2 agonists, inhaled long-acting β_2 agonists, anti-leukotrienes, the cromone nonsteroid inhaled anti-inflammatory drugs cromoglycate and nedocromil, theophylline, oral β_2 agonists and, in the laboratory, inhaled furosemide and heparin. Anticholinergics and antihistamines at conventional doses do not give clinically important protection.

NOCTURNAL ASTHMA

Nocturnal asthma is another clinical syndrome which usually represents an expression of poor asthma control. Up to 40% of apparently stable patients may have sleep disturbance every night and even higher percentages have symptoms more than one night each week. As this is not always volunteered it is important to enquire specifically regarding symptoms at night or first thing in the morning. Furthermore, nocturnal symptoms are also common presenting features in previously undiagnosed asthma. Nocturnal asthma is associated with daytime morbidity, and asthma deaths, including respiratory arrests on ventilators, peak at night.

The mechanisms of nocturnal worsening of asthma are complex but almost certainly involve a variety of circadian (24 hour) biorhythms, including reduction in circulating adrenaline and cortisol, fall in body temperature, increased vagal parasympathetic tone, increased nonspecific airway responsiveness at night, and increased inflammatory responses, including airway eosinophilia and neutrophilia. Other factors include posture, occupational exposures, shift work, exposure to allergens in the home, and timing of medication.

Adequate inhaled steroid therapy is the cornerstone of management. Specific treatments include bedtime administration of inhaled short-acting and, particularly, long-acting β_2 agonists, oral slow-release theophylline preparations, anti-leukotrienes, and oral β_2 agonists. New nocturnal symptoms in the context of unstable asthma may herald the onset of an acute exacerbation indicating a need for a short course of prednisolone. Clinical management also involves attention to other common nocturnal problems, e.g. rhinosinusitis, gastro-oesophageal reflux, and sleep apnoea.

OCCUPATIONAL ASTHMA

Occupational asthma is defined in terms of variable airflow obstruction and/or bronchial hyper-responsiveness caused by an occupational environment and not by stimuli outside the workplace. It is classified depending on whether or not there is a latency period. The usual form develops after a latency period (may be months to years) required for sensitization. The other form develops, without a latency period, after exposure to high concentrations of an irritant, e.g. chlorine or ammonia after an industrial accident. This is known as reactive airways dysfunction syndrome (RADS).

Occupational asthma may account for 5–10% of adult-onset asthma. It is now the commonest industrial lung disease, with an ever increasing list of reported causes (currently > 400). Examples are shown in *Table 25*. It is very important to think of this in every patient, because asthma may potentially be curable if the patient is promptly removed from exposure, but becomes irreversible over time. Removing people from work is a major intervention socially and financially. Occupational asthma is a notifiable condition and the patient may be entitled to compensation. There may be a need to screen others in the workplace.

Pathogenesis

The exact immunological mechanisms are often unclear, though IgE may be implicated with agents classified as high molecular weight (HMW) compounds (such as proteins and polysaccharides) and low molecular weight (LMW) compounds (such as platinum salts or acid anhydrides). Other agents act as haptens, e.g. trimellitic anhydride, requiring conjugation with proteins to become allergenic. Other LMW compounds, such as isocyanates, plicatic acid, and nickel, probably involve cell-mediated immunity with activation of T-lymphocytes and eosinophils and even neutrophils. The extent and duration of exposure are important determinants, but atopy and bronchial responsiveness are of variable significance, as is smoking, human leucocyte antigen (HLA) status, and co-factors, such as viral infection or concomitant exposures.

Table 25 Occupations associated with occupational asthma

High molecular weight agents

Examples of occupation	Source	Agent
Farmers	Grain mites	Insect antigens
Lab workers	Locusts	
Bakers, millers	Wheat, rye, gluten	Plant proteins
Mushroom workers	Mushrooms	
Printers, carpet makers	Gums	Acacia, guar
Lab technicians	Mice, rats	Urine proteins
Vets	Mammals	Cat, dog antigens,
Nurses, doctors	Latex gloves	Latex
Hairdressers	Henna	Conchiolin (?)
Detergent industry	Biological enzymes	*Bacillus subtilis*
Pharmaceuticals		Papain, pepsin
Seafood processors	Seafood	Prawn, crab, oyster antigens
Plumbers	Solder	Aminoethylethanolamine

Low molecular weight agents

Examples of occupation	Source	Agent
IgE-dependent:		
Glue, paint, varnish, and plastics workers	Epoxy resins	Phthalic anhydrides
Platinum workers	Platinum salts	Platinum halides
Metal grinding	Cobalt	
Metal plating	Nickel	
IgE-independent:		
Painters, varnishers	Paint, varnish	Isocyanates (TDI, MDI, HDI, PPI)
Electronics	Solder flux	Colophony
Carpentry, saw mill	Western red cedar	*Thuja plicata*
Wood carvers	Californian redwood	*Sequoia*
Pharmaceuticals	Drugs	Penicillins and so on

Diagnosis

It is important to question all adults with asthma about possible causal or exacerbating agents at work. Established asthmatics with aggravation of symptoms by dust or fumes at work should be distinguished from new asthmatics or even previous asthmatics additionally sensitized to an occupational agent. Enquiries as to whether the patient is better or worse at work, at weekends, or on holiday should be made. There may be associated rhinitis, conjunctivitis, eczema or urticaria. Close enquiry about relevant exposures, lists of hazardous materials, protective equipment, and timing of symptoms must be made.

Investigation centres around confirming asthma (serial PEF, FEV_1, and reversibility) but also confirming the relationship with workplace exposures and finally identifying the specific cause. PEF measurements should be made every 2 hours from waking to sleeping over a period of 4 weeks. Alternatively, non-specific bronchial responsiveness can be measured while at work and then after a period away. This is less sensitive and less specific. Identifying a specific cause may be more difficult, and expert help is usually necessary. Specific IgE measurement or skin testing may be helpful but specific bronchial provocation testing with appropriate controls is the gold standard. Increase in induced sputum eosinophils after occupational exposure may help to confirm the diagnosis.

Management

Several studies have shown that prognosis is worse if patients remain exposed for more than 1 year after symptoms develop. However premature advice to leave work is not advisable. Relations with management may be sensitive but they may be helpful in removing the cause or re-deploying the worker. After removal from exposure improvement in FEV_1 may occur over 12 months while bronchial responsiveness may improve over 2 years. Assessment of long-term disability should therefore be delayed at least 2 years. RADS is diagnosed clinically with compatible physiological measurements, including non-specific bronchial responsiveness. Low-level exposure to the causative agent may be tolerated without problems. The prognosis is variable but is usually good.

PULMONARY EOSINOPHILIA

Pulmonary eosinophilia is a syndrome comprising marked blood eosinophilia (*Table 23*, page 61) and lung tissue eosinophilia usually characterized only by infiltrates on chest radiograph (typically peripheral opacities on HRCT scan). The commonest identifiable cause in the UK is an allergic response to the fungus *Aspergillus fumigatus*, but other causes are commoner in other parts of the world (cf tropical eosinophilia). Many drugs can also induce the syndrome.

ALLERGIC BRONCHOPULMONARY ASPERGILLOSIS

Allergic bronchopulmonary aspergillosis (ABPA) is one manifestation of disease related to *Aspergillus* species, most commonly *A. fumigatus*. Inhalation of the spores of this ubiquitously distributed fungus, commonly found in soil, leads to proliferation in the bronchial tree. Type 1 and type 3 hypersensitivity responses which, in particular individuals, produce high-titre IgE (and IgG) antibodies producing immune complex damage in association with intense eosinophilic infiltration. Mucus plugs heavily infiltrated with eosinophils and fungal hyphae cause proximal bronchial obstruction and distal collapse, eventually leading to central bronchiectasis.

Diagnosis

ABPA occurs in 1–6% of all asthmatics but represents perhaps 10% of severe asthma. There is a spectrum of disease but clinical features include:

❑ Asthma (> 95% of patients).
❑ Eosinophilia ($1.0–3.0 \times 10^9$/l).
❑ Recurrent pulmonary infiltrates (which may be asymptomatic).
❑ IgE response:
  – positive prick skin tests (approx. 100%).
  – high titre radioallergosorbent test (RAST).
❑ IgG precipitins:
  – positive in 70% +.
❑ Elevated total circulating IgE (usually > 1000 IU/l).
❑ *Aspergillus fumigatus* (usually) isolated in sputum.
❑ Bronchial casts or plugs produced.
❑ Central bronchiectasis.

Chest radiographs typically show fleeting shadows, sometimes perihilar infiltrates, segmental collapse/consolidation or 'finger in glove' (bronchocoeles). In advanced cases, bronchiectasis is seen (best shown by HRCT).

Management

Low-dose inhaled steroids have been shown to be ineffective in preventing bronchiectasis, and in many patients severe asthma requires oral corticosteroid therapy. Exacerbations require prednisolone 30 mg or more for 2 weeks with monitoring of lung function and chest radiograph. In addition to conventional management itraconazole 200 mg twice daily for 4–8 months has been shown to be of some benefit in a double-blind, placebo-controlled trial.

CHURG–STRAUSS SYNDROME

Churg–Strauss syndrome (CSS) is one of the systemic vasculitides characterized by asthma, marked eosinophilia (> 1500×10^9/l), and sometimes pulmonary infiltrates. Often there is evidence of other tissue involvement, particularly skin, peripheral nerves, heart, and muscle, with small-vessel necrotizing vasculitis. A pANCA (antineutrophil cytoplasmic antibody) by nuclear immunofluorescence or a positive titre of anti-MPO (myeloperoxidase) antibody occurs in approximately 70% of patients. There may be overlap with other vasculitic syndromes, particularly Wegener's, or microscopic polyarteritis, but diagnosis is clinical. Biopsy evidence of classical granulomatous involvement is rarely obtained. Treatment is urgent because of possible life-threatening complications. High-dose prednisolone is employed first-line followed usually by a course of cyclophosphamide and subsequently azathioprine as adjunctive immunosuppression (also steroid sparing). The prognosis is generally better than for some of the other vasculitides.

CSS has recently been recognized in association with drugs, particularly the leukotriene receptor antagonists (LTRAs), montelukast and zafirlukast. It seems likely that, in the vast majority of cases, patients presented after the reduction of oral steroid therapy (consequent upon the introduction of LTRAs) uncovered pre-existing CSS.

ASPIRIN-INDUCED ASTHMA

Aspirin-induced asthma (AIA) is an acquired syndrome consisting of:

❑ Rhinitis with nasal polyps.
❑ Sinusitis.
❑ Nonatopic asthma.
❑ Aspirin intolerance.

It is commoner in middle-aged women and is associated with eosinophilia.

Aspirin intolerance is shared with intolerance to unselective NSAIDs but not the inducible cyclo-oxygenase-2 (COX-2) inhibitors. It is characterized by cough, wheeze, tightness, ocular injection, nasal blockage, rhinorrhoea, and sometimes rash, sweating, and flushing, occurring 2 minutes to 2 hours after ingestion. Aspirin-induced anaphylaxis is a distinct possibility. Hydrocortisone succinate-induced asthma may coexist with AIA in some patients.

The prevalence of AIA is estimated at 2–5% of patients with asthma by history, but about 10% are positive on challenge. AIA tends to be severe and difficult to manage and the increasing use of NSAIDs makes this an important syndrome.

The pathogenesis of AIA remains unclear. Provoking agents all inhibit cyclo-oxygenase (COX 1 and 2) pathways which lead to the formation of prostaglandins and thromboxane, but paracetamol is safe. There is evidence of overproduction of, and hypersensitivity to, leukotrienes in AIA, and anti-leukotriene drugs block acute reactions and are useful in treatment. There is also evidence of over-expression of epithelial leukotriene synthase in AIA. However, a simple unifying explanation remains elusive.

Management

A high index of suspicion is essential, as avoidance is the key to management. Diagnostic challenge is rarely employed in routine practice. Desensitization has been successfully employed but is rarely used. Treatment follows the general strategies. High-dose inhaled corticosteroids, including to the nose, are the cornerstone of treatment. An early trial of a LTRA is indicated.

ASTHMA IN PREGNANCY

Asthma can occur in pregnancy, and asthmatic patients may need special care in pregnancy. Asthma is most often worse in the third trimester and occasionally very severe after delivery but, fortunately, is extremely rare in labour. The outcome of pregnancy is good if asthma is controlled, but uncontrolled asthma carries major risks to mother and baby.

The need for regular therapy of the mother in pregnancy is always emotive. However, the evidence is clear: inhaled β_2 agonists and inhaled steroids are safe in pregnancy as are oral theophyllines. Salmeterol is also thought to be safe. Oral steroids were initially thought to be associated with cleft palate but subsequent studies have concluded that this is not so. Oral steroids are particularly important in severe asthma and should be used as normal throughout pregnancy. LTRAs are contraindicated at present. Acute asthma should be treated aggressively along the usual lines.

Severe asthma in labour is very rare, but if it occurs standard pain relief should be used. Caesarean section is reserved for standard obstetric indications. Regional block is preferred to general anaesthesia as far as possible. Prostaglandin (PG) E2 is safe in inducing labour, whereas PGF2-alpha (for postpartum haemorrhage) may cause bronchoconstriction and should be avoided. Pregnant mothers and expectant fathers should be strongly discouraged from smoking – including postnatally – because of many adverse effects on the infant's lung function and increased susceptibility to wheeze.

Breast feeding

Breast feeding should be encouraged and may reduce the risk of asthma and wheezing illnesses in children. Very atopic families should be advised to avoid furry pets. None of the inhaled medications, theophylline or prednisolone is contraindicated by breast feeding since drug concentrations are very low in breast milk. Modified milk formulae have not been shown to be beneficial compared with conventional formulae.

PREMENSTRUAL ASTHMA

Premenstrual exacerbation is common in severe asthma, possibly relating to large rapid fluctuations in hormonal state. Conventional management is employed, though one study showed benefit from high-dose intramuscular progesterone.

ACUTE SEVERE ASTHMA

Acute severe asthma is largely preventable as symptoms have usually been present for days beforehand (> 48 hours in > 80% patients). However, once it presents it constitutes a potentially life-threatening medical emergency. The priority is rapidly assessing severity while reassuring the patient and administering oxygen. Objective measures are essential: heart rate, respiratory rate, PEF, oxygen saturation, and determination of arterial blood gases if SaO_2 is below 92% on air (*Table 26*). Patients with life-threatening asthma may not appear distressed and may not show all the features listed.

Hospital referral

Hospital referral is indicated for any patient with features of acute severe or life-threatening asthma, or for more complete assessment because of comorbidites or social circumstances.

Investigations

Chest radiography is not indicated in all patients with acute severe asthma but is performed in all patients with life-threatening asthma or if a complication, such as pneumothorax or pneumonia, is suspected. Arterial blood gases analysis is unpleasant and unpopular with patients but is indicated if SaO_2 is less than 92% on air or if the patient requires oxygen. If

hospital admission is indicated then a full blood count should be routine to exclude anaemia (a raised neutrophil count does not necessarily indicate infection and the eosinophil count is often raised). Biochemical profile is routinely requested under these circumstances, as dehydration and hypokalaemia are common and the latter may be worsened by asthma therapy. C-reactive protein (CRP) determination is reasonable as marked elevation is likely to indicate bacterial infection and the need for antibiotics.

Emergency management

The key aspects of management of acute severe asthma are:
- ❏ Reassurance of the patient.
- ❏ Rapid administration of high-dose inhaled β_2 agonists.
- ❏ Administration of oxygen.
- ❏ Early administration of oral or systemic corticosteroids.

Management in A & E is summarized (**51**).

Table 26 Severity assessment in acute asthma	
Moderate asthma exacerbation	Increasing symptoms Peak expiratory flow (PEF) > 50–75% best or predicted No features of acute severe asthma
Acute severe asthma	Any one of: PEF < 33% best or predicted Respiratory rate > 25 breaths/min Heart rate >110 beats/min Inability to complete sentences in one breath
Life-threatening asthma	Acute severe asthma with any one of: PEF < 33% best or predicted Bradycardia SaO_2 < 92% Dysrhythmia PaO_2 < 8 kPa Hypotension Normal $PaCO_2$ (4.6–6.0 kPa) Exhaustion Silent chest Confusion Cyanosis Coma Feeble respiratory effort
Near fatal asthma	Raised $PaCO_2$ (> 6.0 kPa) and/or requiring mechanical ventilation (with raised inflation pressures)

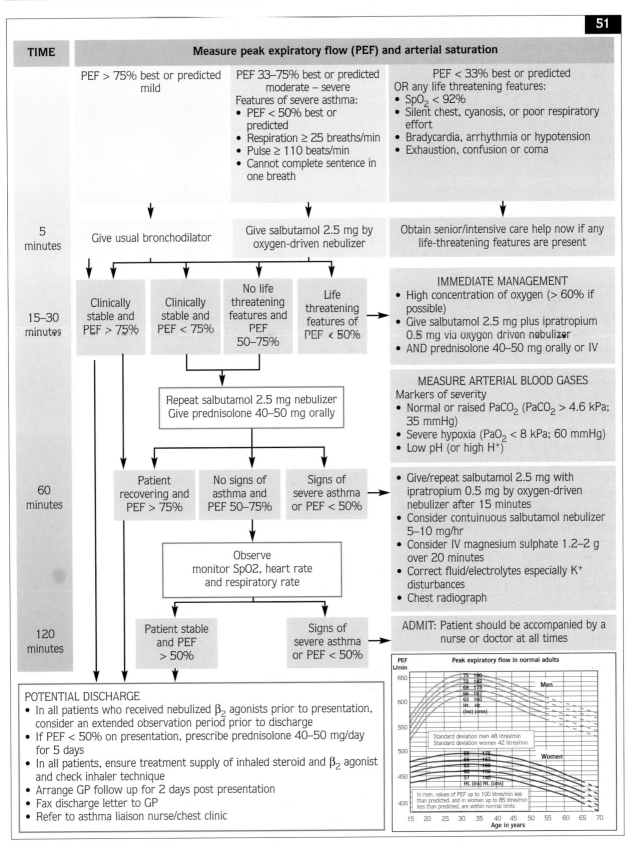

51

TIME	Measure peak expiratory flow (PEF) and arterial saturation

PEF > 75% best or predicted
mild

PEF 33–75% best or predicted
moderate – severe
Features of severe asthma:
- PEF < 50% best or predicted
- Respiration ≥ 25 breaths/min
- Pulse ≥ 110 beats/min
- Cannot complete sentence in one breath

PEF < 33% best or predicted
OR any life threatening features:
- SpO_2 < 92%
- Silent chest, cyanosis, or poor respiratory effort
- Bradycardia, arrhythmia or hypotension
- Exhaustion, confusion or coma

5 minutes

Give usual bronchodilator

Give salbutamol 2.5 mg by oxygen-driven nebulizer

Obtain senior/intensive care help now if any life-threatening features are present

15–30 minutes

Clinically stable and PEF > 75%

Clinically stable and PEF < 75%

No life threatening features and PEF 50–75%

Life threatening features of PEF < 50%

IMMEDIATE MANAGEMENT
- High concentration of oxygen (> 60% if possible)
- Give salbutamol 2.5 mg plus ipratropium 0.5 mg via oxygen driven nebulizer
- AND prednisolone 40–50 mg orally or IV

Repeat salbutamol 2.5 mg nebulizer
Give prednisolone 40–50 mg orally

MEASURE ARTERIAL BLOOD GASES
Markers of severity
- Normal or raised $PaCO_2$ ($PaCO_2$ > 4.6 kPa; 35 mmHg)
- Severe hypoxia (PaO_2 < 8 kPa; 60 mmHg)
- Low pH (or high H^+)

60 minutes

Patient recovering and PEF > 75%

No signs of asthma and PEF 50–75%

Signs of severe asthma or PEF < 50%

- Give/repeat salbutamol 2.5 mg with ipratropium 0.5 mg by oxygen-driven nebulizer after 15 minutes
- Consider continuous salbutamol nebulizer 5–10 mg/hr
- Consider IV magnesium sulphate 1.2–2 g over 20 minutes
- Correct fluid/electrolytes especially K^+ disturbances
- Chest radiograph

Observe
monitor SpO2, heart rate and respiratory rate

120 minutes

Patient stable and PEF > 50%

Signs of severe asthma or PEF < 50%

ADMIT: Patient should be accompanied by a nurse or doctor at all times

POTENTIAL DISCHARGE
- In all patients who received nebulized β_2 agonists prior to presentation, consider an extended observation period prior to discharge
- If PEF < 50% on presentation, prescribe prednisolone 40–50 mg/day for 5 days
- In all patients, ensure treatment supply of inhaled steroid and β_2 agonist and check inhaler technique
- Arrange GP follow up for 2 days post presentation
- Fax discharge letter to GP
- Refer to asthma liaison nurse/chest clinic

51 Management of acute severe asthma in adults in A&E

Bronchodilators

Bronchodilatation is the essential initial aim of treatment and high-dose β_2 agonists are the preferred choice. Salbutamol or terbutaline can be given using a large volume spacer, which in studies have been shown to equally as effective as nebulization, which is nevertheless widely used. Nebulizers should be driven at 6–8 l/min, preferably using oxygen (to prevent worsening hypoxaemia), in hospital or in the ambulance. At home or in the surgery it is more important to give the β_2 agonist urgently rather than worry about the absence of supplemental oxygen. It is better to give salbutamol 2.5 mg frequently rather than 5 mg 4-hourly, and continuous nebulization is sometimes required. Nebulized ipratropium bromide 0.5 mg 4–6-hourly is recommended in acute severe or life-threatening asthma or if there is a poor initial response to β_2 agonists.

Intravenous therapy

Intravenous (IV) therapy is rarely required but re-hydration or correction of hypokalaemia is sometimes necessary. A single dose of magnesium 1.2–2.0 G as an IV infusion over 20 minutes has been shown to be safe and effective in rapidly increasing FEV_1 in acute severe asthma.

Intravenous aminophylline is not recommended routinely but it may be indicated in very severe asthma as a loading dose of 5 mg/kg body weight over 20 minutes unless the patient is already on maintenance oral therapy. In such cases the theophylline level should be measured urgently. Maintenance infusion is at a rate of 0.5–0.7 mg/kg body weight/hour and theophylline levels should be checked daily because of potential serious side-effects. Intravenous β_2 agonists are rarely indicated and should only be given with electrocardiogram (ECG) monitoring.

Oxygen

High-flow (40–60%) inspired oxygen by Hudson mask is usually adequate to achieve $SaO_2 > 92\%$. Unlike in COPD oxygen administration is very unlikely to precipitate hypercapnia. Blood gases are only indicated if SaO_2 is < 92% on air or if the patient is exhausted. The usual picture in acute asthma is of a low PaO_2 and a low $PaCO_2$. A normal $PaCO_2$ on presentation should raise concern that it is increasing and that mechanical ventilation may become necessary.

Steroids

Prednisolone 30–50 mg orally is preferred as long as patients are able to swallow and retain tablets. If there is any suspicion of poor absorption, e.g. in a patient on ITU, hydrocortisone 100 mg 6-hourly is adequate (higher doses are likely to cause myopathy). Oral steroids can be stopped abruptly provided high-dose inhaled steroids have been introduced beforehand and provided patients are not steroid dependent and do not have brittle asthma or frequent courses of steroids.

Antibiotics

Antibiotics are overused and are not indicated routinely in acute asthma but may be used if there is chest radiograph shadowing, raised CRP or high fever.

Hospital admission

Hospital admission is indicated in patients with life-threatening or near fatal asthma (*Table 26*, page 72), when severe asthma is present (PEF is < 75% best or predicted) 1 hour after initial therapy, or because of previous near fatal or brittle asthma, persisting severe symptoms, exacerbation despite adequate prednisolone, presentation at night, pregnancy, concerns about compliance, living alone, social isolation, psychological problems, or learning or physical disability.

Intensive care

Admission to ITU is indicated if the patient is not improving despite therapy, particularly in cases of:
❏ Falling PEF.
❏ Rising heart rate.
❏ Persisting or worsening hypoxaemia.
❏ Rising $PaCO_2$ or H^+ concentration or falling pH.
❏ Exhaustion.
❏ Confusion, drowsiness or coma.
❏ Respiratory arrest.

Intubation may be difficult, carries significant risk, and should be performed in the ITU by an experienced anaesthetist. Mechanical ventilation is associated with a variety of complications but is usually life-saving. Noninvasive ventilation should not be used in asthma.

Discharge from hospital

Planned discharge should occur once nebulizer therapy has been discontinued for at least 24 hours, PEF is > 75% best or predicted, ideally with PEF diurnal variability < 25%, and patients have inhalers that they are able to use satisfactorily, some form of agreed action plan, and a follow-up asthma clinic appointment.

Checklist after the acute attack

Every attack of asthma or emergency attendance represents a failure, to some extent, of previous asthma management. Therefore, after an attack the opportunity must be taken to address various issues to reduce the risk of future exacerbations. These factors are listed in *Table 27*. Near-fatal asthma requires life-long specialist follow up. In one series nearly a quarter of patients were dead within 8 years of mechanical ventilation for acute severe asthma.

BRITTLE ASTHMA

Brittle asthma is divided into two types:
- ❏ Type 1 patients show wide PEF variability (> 40% diurnal variation for > 50% of the time, over a period of > 150 days despite intensive therapy).
- ❏ Type 2 patients suffer sudden severe exacerbations against a background of apparently well controlled asthma.

The mechanisms involved in both types are unclear. Management of both generally involves continuous oral steroids because of the concern regarding sudden death. In type 1 subcutaneous infusion of terbutaline may be helpful. Self-administration of parenteral adrenaline may be helpful in type 2 patients, though its half-life is very short.

ASTHMA DEATH

Death due to asthma is a catastrophe which continues to occur but which, in over 70% of cases, remains preventable. Confidential enquiries into death from asthma have repeatedly shown that death is due to under-appreciation of asthma severity (without objective measurement of airway diameter, e.g. PEF), under-usage of oral steroids, overuse of inhaled β_2 agonists, and delay. It occurs from hypoxia and is a very rare event if the patient reaches hospital breathing spontaneously. This is because mechanical ventilation is life saving and in most cases the pathophysiology can be reversed within a few days using systemic steroids. Particular attention should be paid to patients with several risk factors for asthma death (*Table 28*).

Table 27 Checklist for use after an emergency attendance or admission

Was this potentially fatal asthma?
- ❏ If so, the patient requires lifelong specialist follow-up

Is the patient's inhaler technique satisfactory?
- ❏ Check technique, re-educate or change inhaler device

Was the patient prescribed/taking adequate preventer therapy?
- ❏ Ask about adherence, elicit problems or fears, and re-educate

Was there an avoidable precipitating cause?
- ❏ Check possible triggers (*Table 20*, page 59) especially NSAIDs or β-blockers (including eye drops)

Was this a genuine sudden severe (brittle) attack?
- ❏ Advise specialist care, e.g. self-administration of parenteral adrenaline

Is the patient a 'poor perceiver'?
- ❏ Encourage PEF monitoring

Did the patient respond appropriately to the exacerbation?

Did the patient have a written personal action plan?
- ❏ Explain and produce an individualized action plan

Table 28 Risk factors for asthma death

- ❏ Female sex
- ❏ Long-standing asthma
- ❏ Overuse of β_2 agonists
- ❏ 'Brittle asthma' (marked PEF fluctuation)
- ❏ Steroid-dependent asthma
- ❏ Previous admission with very severe (near fatal) asthma
- ❏ Aspirin-induced asthma
- ❏ Fungal-sensitive asthma
- ❏ Psychosocial problems
- ❏ Use of psychoactive medication
- ❏ Poor understanding of disease
- ❏ Poor compliance with medication and follow-up

DIFFICULT ASTHMA

Difficult asthma has been defined as asthma resistant to standard therapy (> 2,000 μg of BDP equivalent daily together with other treatment).

STEROID-DEPENDENT ASTHMA

By definition this is severe asthma where, despite all other therapeutic measures, including maximum inhaled corticosteroid doses, patients cannot be weaned from maintenance oral corticosteroid. These patients are disproportionately important; they suffer severe disability from their disease (*Table 22*, page 60) and from the treatment (*Table 24*, page 64). In addition 10% of the most severe patients incur 50% of total asthma costs.

These patients require long-term specialist follow-up. The diagnosis must be confirmed as far as possible. Attention is given to excluding or treating associated conditions – rhinosinusitis, gastro-oesophageal reflux, hyperventilation, and anxiety and/or depression. In addition, complications of steroid therapy must be monitored and treated – obesity, hypertension, osteoporosis, cataracts, glaucoma, and growth (in children). In smokers, smoking cessation measures are vital.

STEROID-SPARING THERAPY

Steroid-sparing immunosuppressive agents with evidence of efficacy include:

❏ Methotrexate.
❏ Cyclosporin.
❏ Oral gold.

A trial of 3-month therapy is justified and modest effects are seen in 'responders'. Unfortunately benefit does not usually persist after treatment is stopped and side-effects require careful monitoring.

Corticosteroid resistance

A small number of patients with corticosteroid resistance have been described. It remains unclear how common this is or whether it represents one end of a continuous spectrum of response to oral steroids. The definition requires demonstration of the acute bronchodilator effect of a β_2 agonist with minimal response to a 2-week course of oral prednisolone. It is important to exclude misdiagnosis, poor compliance, and inadequate treatment of rhinosinusitis and gastro-oesophageal reflux.

Different mechanisms have been described, ranging from primary corticosteroid receptor abnormalities to specific defects in lymphocyte or monocyte steroid receptor response *in vitro* and *in vivo*, e.g. increased activity of the specific transcription factor activated peptide-1 (AP-1). It is important to appreciate that steroid-resistant asthmatics remain susceptible to steroid-induced side-effects.

Chapter 8 Diffuse parenchymal (interstitial) lung disease

INTRODUCTION

Diffuse parenchymal lung disease (DPLD), or interstitial lung disease, denotes around 200 conditions characterized by pathology mainly affecting the lung interstitium (as opposed to respiratory pathology affecting the airways, such as in asthma and COPD). This group of diseases generates considerable diagnostic and therapeutic uncertainty, but precise diagnosis is important in determining prognosis and optimum treatment.

DPLD may be acute or chronic, associated with occupational dust inhalation, leisure activities or drug exposure, related to infection or systemic conditions, or arise for no obvious cause. Classification can be somewhat daunting; a simple outline of the more common conditions is given in *Table 29*. This chapter will focus on the more frequently encountered conditions, including sarcoidosis, cryptogenic fibrosing alveolitis (CFA), occupational and recreational DPLD, DPLD associated with collagen vascular disease, and drug-induced disease. Details of some of the more unusual conditions that may occasionally be encountered are provided at the end of this chapter.

The last two decades of the twentieth century saw a significant increase in knowledge and recognition of DPLD. This resulted in part from the advent and widespread use of high-resolution computed tomography (HRCT), and re-evaluation of histopathological patterns by lung pathologists. Furthermore, the relative absence of effective treatments promoted research aimed at increasing understanding of the mechanisms underlying pathogenesis. New and more effective therapies are now being explored and tested in clinical trials.

SARCOIDOSIS

EPIDEMIOLOGY

Sarcoidosis is the commonest DPLD, occurs worldwide, and affects both sexes and all races. It typically affects adults between the ages of 20 and 40 years. The putative incidence varies substantially worldwide, partly because of different prevalence in different ethnic groups and partly because it is unrecognized in many countries. Prevalence varies between 3 (in Caucasian populations) and 47 (in African American populations) per 100,000 in North America, and rises to 64 per 100,000 in Scandinavia. In addition to being more commonly affected, Blacks and Afro-Caribbeans suffer more severe disease. In 1999 there were 115 deaths from sarcoidosis in Great Britain, mortality typically being due to progressive respiratory failure or central nervous system or myocardial involvement.

The first description of sarcoidosis is attributed to an English physician, Jonathon Hutchinson, in 1877, but its aetiology remains unknown. It has long been suspected that a specific causative agent exists, such as a micro-organism, but none has been proven. Genetic factors are thought to influence susceptibility to the disease and/or prognosis in affected individuals.

PATHOGENESIS AND PATHOLOGY

Histologically, sarcoidosis is characterized by noncaseating granulomas (in the absence of acid-fast bacilli indicating tuberculosis) in affected organs. The accumulating T-cells usually bear the helper CD4 phenotype and release cytokines, including interferon-γ and interleukin-2. Sarcoid alveolar macrophages also produce various cytokines, including tumour necrosis factor α. Sarcoidosis may affect any organ, but the lungs are involved in over 90% of patients.

Table 29 Outline classification of commoner diffuse parenchymal lung diseases

Known cause

❑ Drugs or radiation

❑ Occupational (pneumoconiosis, extrinsic allergic alveolitis)

❑ Collagen vascular disease

❑ Lymphangitis carcinomatosis

❑ Infection (e.g. human immunodeficiency virus, *Mycoplasma*)

Unknown cause

❑ Cryptogenic fibrosing alveolitis (usual interstitial pneumonia)

❑ Other idiopathic interstitial pneumonias

Granulomatous

❑ Sarcoidosis

CLINICAL FEATURES

The commonest manifestation of thoracic sarcoidosis is bilateral hilar lymphadenopathy (BHL) as seen on the chest radiograph (52). In some patients it is asymptomatic and detected on a routine radiograph performed for other purposes. In others it may present with cough, breathlessness, erythema nodosum, fatigue, fever or indeed pyrexia of unknown origin (PUO), arthralgia, or a combination of any of these features. Interstitial lung involvement may be asymptomatic and physical signs absent, but breathlessness may develop. Haemoptysis and finger clubbing are rare and lung crackles are present in fewer than 20% of patients.

Extrathoracic sarcoidosis typically affects the skin, eyes, bones, heart, nervous system or kidneys (*Table 30*). Skin lesions include erythema nodosum (53), nodules, lupus pernio, and scar infiltration (54). Eye disease can manifest as lacrimal gland enlargement (55), or as anterior or posterior uveitis. Posterior uveitis is the main cause of loss of vision and requires urgent treatment.

Table 30 Extrathoracic sarcoidosis

Affected organ	Frequency
Lymphoid system	Palpable peripheral lymph nodes in 33%
Heart	Myocardial involvement in 5%
Liver	Granulomas in 50–80%
Skin	25%
Ocular lesions	11–83%; uveitis most frequent
Nervous system	< 10%
Musculoskeletsal system	Arthralgia in 25–39%
Gastrointestinal tract	< 1%
Haematological manifestations	Mild leucopenia in up to 10%; mild anaemia in 4–20%
Parotid glands	Parotitis in < 6%
Endocrine manifestations	Hypercalcaemia in 2–10%
Reproductive organs	Rare and usually asymptomatic
Renal tract	Rarely interstitial nephritis

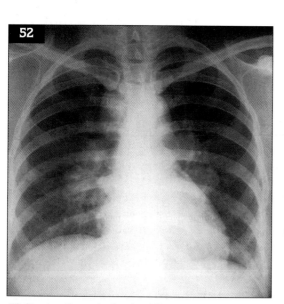

52 Chest radiograph showing bilateral hilar lymphadenopathy in sarcoidosis. The differential diagnosis of these appearances includes tuberculosis and lymphoma. It is important to exclude these conditions before making a diagnosis of sarcoidosis

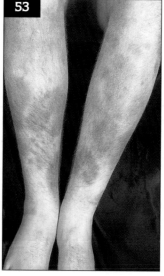

53 Erythema nodosum in sarcoidosis

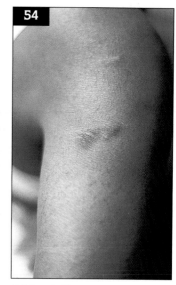

54 Scar infiltration in sarcoidosis

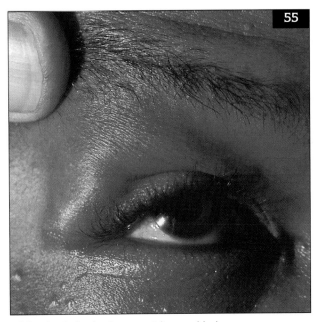

55 Lacrimal gland enlargement in sarcoidosis

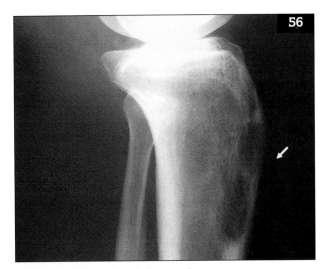

56 Bone cyst in sarcoidosis (arrowed)

Table 31 Chest radiograph staging of sarcoidosis

Stage	Finding
0	Normal chest radiograph
I	Bilateral hilar lymphadenopathy (BHL)
II	BHL and pulmonary infiltrates
III	Pulmonary infiltrates without BHL
IV	Pulmonary fibrosis

Bone and joint disease includes dactylitis, osteopenic lesions (**56**), and arthralgia. Deforming arthritis is rare. Granulomas affecting the heart and conducting system can cause conduction defects, including third degree heart block and cardiomyopathy. Nervous system involvement may manifest as cranial and/or peripheral nerve palsies, commonly a VIIth nerve palsy, space occupying lesions which can result in seizures or diffuse CNS disease, granulomatous meningitis, or pituitary disease causing diabetes insipidus. The kidneys may be affected by hypercalcaemic nephropathy and renal calculi, or rarely, interstitial nephritis.

INVESTIGATIONS AND DIAGNOSIS

Sarcoidosis is diagnosed on the basis of clinical symptoms and signs and on the results of investigations. There is no single diagnostic test for sarcoidosis, and no one good test exists for monitoring disease activity thereafter. Particular attention must therefore be paid to the history and examination, both at presentation and at subsequent clinic visits.

Routine blood tests include full blood count, biochemical screen, including corrected calcium and inflammatory markers, including erythrocyte sedimentation rate (ESR) and C-reactive protein (CRP). Mild leucopenia is common, mild anaemia may be present, and inflammatory markers may be raised. The chest radiograph may be normal, or show BHL, BHL with infiltrates, infiltrates alone, or fibrosis. Radiological staging is a guide to prognosis (*Table 31*).

Tuberculin skin testing helps to exclude tuberculosis; it is typically negative in sarcoidosis. A 24-hour urine calcium estimation must be performed to exclude hypercalcuria. Serum angiotensin converting enzyme (ACE) level should be measured, but a mildly raised level is nondiagnostic and in some patients ACE levels are normal at presentation and remain normal throughout the course of the disease. ECG should be performed to exclude heart block.

Full lung function testing is mandatory but must not be performed until open (smear positive) pulmonary tuberculosis is excluded because of the risk of contaminating equipment. Lung function tests may be normal or show a restrictive (small-lung) pattern with reduced gas transfer (DLCO) (see Chapter 4, page 24). Sarcoidosis can, however, also cause airflow obstruction. DLCO must be corrected for haemoglobin concentration, as an anaemia of 10 g/dl will reduce gas transfer by around 15%.

Routine HRCT scanning is not required by

current North American and UK guidelines, but is recommended where there is diagnostic uncertainty, such as concern about the possibility of lymphoma, and is performed routinely in many centres. Typical HRCT features include mediastinal lymphadenopathy, nodules, and beading along bronchovascular bundles and fissures (57).

The Kveim test, an intradermal injection of sarcoid spleen tissue resulting in granulomas at the injection site after 4–6 weeks, is not usually performed in the UK because of possible transmission of infection, including infection by slow viruses.

Gallium scanning is expensive and involves the patient making two hospital visits, one for injection and one for scanning. It involves significant radiation exposure and has limited value in diagnosing sarcoidosis. It is, however, sometimes used to assess disease activity, and to help diagnose sarcoidosis in extrathoracic disease not accessible to biopsy.

Current North American and UK guidelines recommend histological confirmation of the diagnosis. Initially, a bronchoscopy with bronchoalveloar lavage (BAL) and bronchial and transbronchial biopsies is usually performed. Transbronchial biopsy carries a small risk (< 10%) of pneumothorax. Analysis of the cellular constituents of BAL typically reveals a lymphocytosis with increased CD4:CD8 T-cell ratio. Bronchial and/or transbronchial biopsies typically show noncaseating granulomas without evidence of acid-fast bacilli. In some patients granulomas are not detectable

in these small tissue samples and further means of histological confirmation has to be sought. This may involve proceeding to mediastinoscopy or biopsy of skin, lymph node, or other lesions. Biopsy of erythema nodosum is usually not recommended.

MANAGEMENT

The natural history of sarcoidosis is highly variable and disease activity tends to wax and wane, either spontaneously or in response to therapy. In asymptomatic disease with no lung function abnormalities, treatment is not indicated and the patient can be monitored at 3–6 monthly intervals.

In patients with vital organ involvement, including progressive deterioration in lung function, prompt treatment with oral corticosteroids is indicated. The usual starting dose is 20–40 mg of oral prednisolone daily for between 1 and 3 months, with subsequent gradual reduction of the dose to the lowest possible maintenance dose. The usual length of initial treatment is up to 2 years, with around half of those patients who require steroids initially requiring further courses subsequently. Patients must be warned about the common side-effects of systemic corticosteroid treatment, including weight gain, osteoporosis, diabetes, hypertension, and cataracts. A rare but potentially serious complication is avascular necrosis of the hip.

Some patients require additional treatment with alternative immunosuppressants, although there are limited data on their efficacy. Frequently used agents include methotrexate, azathioprine, and hydroxychloroquine. Methotrexate and azathioprine confer a risk of potentially serious side-effects, including bone marrow suppression and teratogenicity. These must be discussed fully with the patient before starting treatment. Monitoring is required as recommended by manufacturers' and national guidelines, and includes, as a minimum, regular full blood count, urea, and electrolytes and liver function tests.

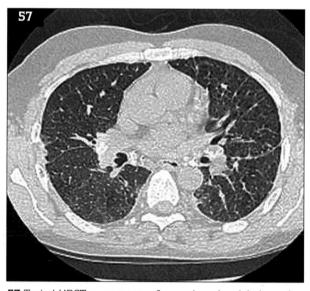

57 Typical HRCT appearances of parenchymal nodularity and bronchovascular beading in sarcoidosis

CASE STUDY

CASE STUDY 1

A 32-year-old woman attends the chest clinic complaining of red, tender lumps over her shins and painful ankles. Closer questioning reveals that she has been feeling unwell for the last 6 weeks with enlarged glands and intermittent fevers. She has a non-productive cough. She recently returned from a trip to visit her family in Pakistan but is not aware of any contact with tuberculosis. Examination reveals a pyrexia of 37.5°C, erythema nodosum, and cervical lymphadenopathy. The chest is clear. Initial investigations reveal abnormal liver function (mild transaminitis) and BHL on chest radiography.

The differential diagnosis includes tuberculosis and sarcoidosis. Lymphoma is less likely; Hodgkin's disease rarely causes erythema nodosum. A Heaf test should be performed. If negative, this supports a diagnosis of sarcoidosis and makes tuberculosis less likely. BAL should be performed and lavage fluid sent to the microbiology laboratory to look for acid-fast bacilli, as well as to cytology for a cell count. If no acid-fast bacilli are found on Ziehl–Neelsen (ZN) stain or after 8 weeks' culture, this makes tuberculosis much less likely. Endobronchial and transbronchial biopsies may reveal noncaseating granulomas typical of sarcoidosis. Finally, HRCT scan may help if it shows parenchymal disease typical of sarcoidosis, but absence of parenchymal disease does not exclude the diagnosis. Lung function testing should not be performed before excluding open (smear positive) tuberculosis as far as possible. Queries about when and how to perform lung function tests should be addressed to the lung function laboratory, and local hospital guidelines strictly followed.

Summary of sarcoidosis

- ❑ It is the commonest DPLD.
- ❑ Prevalence is higher in Blacks and Afro-Caribbeans, who suffer more severe disease.
- ❑ It is a multisystem disease of unknown aetiology; it affects the lungs in over 90% of cases.
- ❑ Biopsy showing noncaseating granulomas in the absence of acid-fast bacilli is required to confirm diagnosis.
- ❑ Patients with vital organ involvement or progressive lung function deterioration require treatment with oral corticosteroids.

CRYPTOGENIC FIBROSING ALVEOLITIS

EPIDEMIOLOGY

Cryptogenic fibrosing alveolitis (CFA), termed idiopathic pulmonary fibrosis (IPF) in North America, affects men about twice as often as women. Patients are typically at least 50 years old when the diagnosis is made. The cause is unclear (hence the term 'cryptogenic'), but numerous triggers have been proposed. Case-control studies suggest that cigarette smoking and exposure to wood or metal dust confer increased risk. Some studies have suggested that infectious agents, such as viruses or small intracellular bacteria, may be implicated, but it remains unclear whether they play a role in pathogenesis. There are no good data on genotypes predisposing to the illness, but current evidence suggests that genetic factors may influence its severity. The condition may be familial.

Recent estimates of prevalence give figures of 13–20 per 100,000 of the population with an incidence of 7–11 per 100,000 per year. The incidence rises steeply with age, being approximately six times more frequent in those aged over 75 than in the age range 55–64. Prognosis is poor despite treatment, with 5-year survival < 25% and median survival of 2.8 years. Respiratory failure and cardiovascular disease are the commonest causes of death, but CFA is also associated with an increased risk of lung cancer.

PATHOGENESIS AND PATHOLOGY

The pathological corollary of clinical CFA is termed usual interstitial pneumonia (UIP), as distinct from other idiopathic interstitial pneumonias (*Table 29*, page 77). These are not dealt with here. UIP is characterized by progressive and patchy interstitial fibrosis with loss of normal lung architecture and honeycomb change. The disease begins at the periphery of the pulmonary lobule and is usually sub-pleural. Fibroblastic foci are typically present at the junction of fibrosis with normal lung, and inflammation is usually mild. Mildly reactive type II cells may be present, indicating ongoing lung injury. Fibrosis is associated with fibroblast activation resulting in enhanced collagen synthesis and deposition.

CLINICAL FEATURES

CFA presents insidiously, patients reporting a nonproductive cough, progressive breathlessness on exertion, and variable degrees of general malaise, weight loss, and arthralgia. The diagnosis requires a high index of suspicion, and a thorough and exhaustive history is essential to rule out conditions that mimic CFA. Particular attention must be paid to drug history, family history, hobbies, bird exposures, and environmental exposures. A history of arthritis (as opposed to mild, nonspecific arthralgia) points away from CFA and towards pulmonary fibrosis associated with collagen vascular disease. Haemoptysis is rare and should raise the suspicion of lung cancer or pulmonary embolism.

Finger clubbing is observed in 25–50% of patients. In > 60% of patients fine ('Velcro') end-inspiratory crackles are heard on auscultation, most prevalent at the lung bases. Careful inspection of the skin is required to rule out other possible causes of DPLD, including sarcoidosis and collagen vascular disease. In advanced cases there may be cyanosis and/or pulmonary hypertension secondary to hypoxaemia. Carbon dioxide retention is uncommon; instead patients may progress to develop type I respiratory failure.

INVESTIGATIONS AND DIAGNOSIS

CFA is a diagnosis of exclusion. Baseline blood tests may reveal a raised ESR and/or hypergamma-globulinaemia. Anti-nuclear antibodies (ANA) and rheumatoid factor are present in up to one third of patients. In early disease, the chest radiograph typically reveals bilateral diffuse nodular or reticulonodular shadowing, most marked at the lung bases (58). HRCT is more sensitive than chest radiograph, thereby allowing earlier diagnosis, and helps to increase the level of confidence in a diagnosis of CFA. Characteristic HRCT findings include bilateral basal interstitial reticular opacities, honeycomb changes, traction bronchiectasis, and volume loss (59).

Lung function tests typically show a restrictive (small-lung) ventilatory defect with reduced transfer factor. In early disease the only abnormality may be a widened alveolar–arterial (A–a) gradient. Unless there is co-existing COPD, CFA is unlikely where lung volumes are preserved or increased.

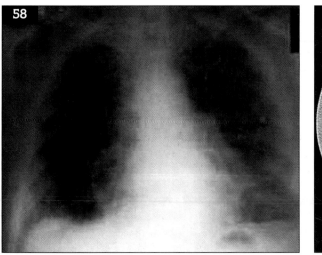

58 Chest radiograph showing bilateral basal reticulonodular shadowing in cryptogenic fibrosing alveolitis

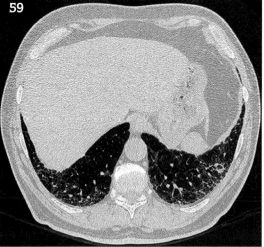

59 High resolution CT showing typical appearances of advanced lung fibrosis with traction bronchiectasis and honeycombing in cryptogenic fibrosing alveolitis

BAL may help exclude an alternative diagnosis. BAL fluid typically shows an increased total cell count with a raised proportion of neutrophils and/or eosinophils. Surgical lung biopsy may be necessary to confirm the diagnosis. It is recommended in suspected CFA when the diagnosis is uncertain, especially when clinical or radiological features are not typical of CFA, provided there are no contraindications to surgery and the potential benefits outweigh the risk. *Table 32* summarizes current North American and European criteria for a diagnosis of CFA.

MANAGEMENT

Corticosteroids and immunosuppressant agents have had little impact on long-term survival in CFA, but are recommended pending discovery of a more effective approach. The appropriateness of therapy in an individual patient will depend on several factors, including the patient's functional status and age. UK guidelines recommend initial treatment with oral prednisolone at a dose of 0.5 mg/kg and azathioprine at 2–3 mg/kg. Patients should be re-assessed at 1 month with a chest radiograph and lung function tests. Response or stability is followed by a slow reduction in prednisolone dose, as this indicates a failure to respond to treatment. A decline should be followed by a more rapid reduction in the dose. Response is defined as an increase in VC and/or TLCO of 10%, and decline by a fall in VC and/or TLCO of 10%. Close monitoring for adverse effects of treatment is mandatory. Alternative treatments include cyclophosphamide and newer

agents in clinical trials. Referral for assessment for lung transplantation may be considered if first-line treatment fails.

Patients in respiratory failure require assessment for long-term oxygen therapy as described in Chapter 6. Current UK guidelines recommend supplemental oxygen in pulmonary fibrosis when resting PaO_2 on air is ≤ 8 kPa.

Table 32 Criteria for a diagnosis of cryptogenic fibrosing alveolitis

Major criteria

❏ Exclusion of other known causes of DPLD (e.g. drug toxicity, environmental exposures, and connective tissue disease)

❏ Abnormal lung function tests including evidence of restriction with impaired gas exchange

❏ Bibasal reticular abnormalities on HRCT

❏ Transbronchial biopsy specimen or BAL fluid showing no features to support an alternative diagnosis

Minor criteria

❏ Age > 50 years

❏ Insidious onset of otherwise unexplained breathlessness on exertion

❏ Duration of illness ≥ 3 months

❏ Bilateral basal inspiratory crackles (dry or 'Velcro' type)

❏ BAL, bronchoalveolar lavage; DPLD, diffuse parenchymal lung disease; HRCT, high resolution computed tomography

---

CASE STUDY

CASE STUDY

A 59-year-old man attends the chest clinic with an 8-year history of slowly worsening breathlessness and dry cough. He can now walk just 200 metres. Past medical history includes recently diagnosed noninsulin dependent diabetes and a perforated peptic ulcer when aged 48. He has worked as an office manager all his life and gave up smoking 2 years ago. There are no birds at home. On examination he is overweight (BMI 28), has finger clubbing, and bilateral fine basal crackles. Chest radiograph performed last month at the request of his general practitioner shows reticulonodular shadowing in both lower lobes.

Question: What initial investigations would you perform?

Initial investigations should include baseline haematology and biochemistry, including inflammatory markers, auto-immune serology, HRCT, and full lung function tests, including spirometry, volumes, and gas transfer factor. Results show normal full blood count, ESR 56 mm/hr, normal biochemical profile excepting a random blood glucose of 23, weakly positive rheumatoid factor and negative ANA. HRCT shows established fibrosis in a basal, sub-pleural distribution typical of CFA. Lung function tests show a restrictive pattern with small lung volumes, reduced gas transfer (TLCO 64% predicted). Oximetry is 98%.

SUMMARY OF CRYPTOGENIC FIBROSING ALVEOLITIS

- ❏ CFA predominantly affects men aged over 50 years (male:female ratio 2:1); the prognosis is poor, with median survival 2.8 years.
- ❏ Links have been established to cigarette smoking and exposure to wood or metal dust.
- ❏ The onset is insidious, with dry cough and breathlessness on exertion of 3 months' duration.
- ❏ Finger clubbing and end-inspiratory 'Velcro' crackles are common.
- ❏ The pathological corollary is usual interstitial pneumonia (UIP).
- ❏ CFA is characterized by progressive and patchy interstitial fibrosis with loss of normal lung architecture and honeycomb change.
- ❏ First-line treatment is with prednisolone and azathioprine.

OCCUPATIONAL AND RECREATIONAL DPLD

DPLD resulting from occupational or recreational pursuits can be divided into those caused by exposure to inhaled inorganic dusts or mineral fibres, and those caused by exposure to inhaled organic dusts. The second group of conditions are referred to collectively as extrinsic allergic alveolitis (EAA) or hypersensitivity pneumonitis. As they have distinct aetiologies and characteristics, the two groups are considered separately.

DPLD DUE TO INHALED INORGANIC DUSTS OR MINERAL FIBRES
Asbestosis

Asbestosis arises from inhaled asbestos fibres. This condition is distinct from the other forms of lung disease caused by asbestos. These include pleural plaques, malignant mesothelioma (see Chapter 9, page 99), and carcinoma of the bronchus (see Chapter 5, page 42). In 1998 there were 165 deaths from asbestosis in the UK. The number of deaths due to occupational lung disease has risen rapidly since the late 1980s, mainly due to a 75% increase in the number of mesothelioma deaths.

Asbestos, a naturally occurring mineral, has unique physical properties. It is resistant to acid, alkali, and heat, and is an excellent and cheap insulating material. It degrades throughout its lifetime by splitting longitudinally into ever smaller fibres, which can be inhaled into the lungs and deposited in terminal bronchioles. Asbestos fibres may be identified in BAL fluid, or in surgical or post-mortem biopsy specimens. Histology reveals interstitial inflammation and fibrosis with or without honeycombing.

There is a latency period of 15–20 years from first exposure to the development of asbestosis. Those at high risk include shipbuilders and construction workers. Patients may present with breathlessness, or the disease may be detected incidentally on a chest radiograph. Crackles are present. Chest radiograph, HRCT, and lung function testing reveal findings similar to those seen in CFA. Diagnosis is based on a consistent history of exposure to asbestos and evidence of interstitial fibrosis. The co-existent finding of pleural plaques, if present, indicating previous asbestos exposure, helps confirm the diagnosis. Histological confirmation is not usually sought and is not recommended by current North American guidelines.

Asbestosis is generally slowly progressive. There is no proven effective therapy and management is supportive. Patients are advised to seek specialist legal advice regarding potential compensation from both government and employer.

Pneumoconiosis

Coal worker's pneumoconiosis (CWP) results from inhalation and deposition of coal dust in the lungs. In simple CWP the chest radiograph shows small rounded opacities only; this condition is asymptomatic and causes no physical signs. Complicated CWP (progressive massive fibrosis) is defined by large opacities on the chest radiograph (2 cm or greater), and clinical and physiological features of interstitial fibrosis similar to those of CFA. This condition contributes to premature morbidity and mortality. In 1999 there were 1,215 deaths from pneumoconiosis in the UK. CWP is diagnosed on the basis of occupational history and chest radiograph findings without recourse to histological confirmation.

Caplan's syndrome denotes a nodular lung reaction in individuals exposed to coal dust who also have rheumatoid arthritis (RA), or who develop RA within the subsequent 5–10 years. There is no proven effective therapy for CWP and management is supportive. Co-existent airflow obstruction is treated as described in Chapter 6, with advice on smoking cessation and correction of hypoxaemia. Improved mining methods should reduce future risk to miners.

Silicosis

Silicosis, recognized since antiquity, denotes a spectrum of pulmonary disease caused by inhaled silica. A wide variety of industries are associated with silicosis. They include gold, tin, iron, copper, nickel, silver, tungsten, uranium, and coal mining. Construction industry workers, especially when tunnelling through rock with high silica content, and those involved in quarrying and stone cutting, or foundry work, are also at risk. Sandblasting, used in ship building and oil-rig maintenance, confers a high risk. Accurate prevalence figures are difficult to obtain because of the many different occupations involved, the participation of transient workers, the variability of disease detection, and differing reporting practices.

Histology typically reveals intrapulmonary 'silicotic' nodules. The central zone is hyalinized and composed of concentrically arranged collagen fibres; the peripheral zone is less organized and contains macrophages, lymphocytes, and lesser amounts of loosely formed collagen. Birefringent particles may be seen under polarized light microscopy.

Mild disease may be asymptomatic or associated with a chronic productive cough due to dust-induced bronchitis. Examination of the chest is usually unremarkable. As the disease progresses, patients may develop breathlessness and ultimately respiratory failure. In these patients breath sounds are diminished because of associated emphysema. Crackles and finger clubbing are not a feature. The chest radiograph typically shows 'eggshell' calcification of hilar lymph nodes together with nodules of various size depending on the stage of the disease. In late disease there may be extensive fibrosis, most prominent in the upper lobes. Lung function tests initially show a restrictive pattern with reduced KCO, but airflow obstruction may develop in parallel with emphysema.

Complications include TB due to impaired cell-mediated immunity, and an increased risk of lung cancer. There is no proven effective treatment and management is supportive.

DPLD DUE TO INHALED ORGANIC DUSTS (EXTRINSIC ALLERGIC ALVEOLITIS)
Epidemiology

The prevalence of extrinsic allergic alveolitis (EAA) varies from country to country and, even within one country, the rate may vary owing to fluctuations in local climate, season, geographical conditions, customs, and the presence of industrial manufacturing plants. The prevalence of EAA is difficult to record accurately because it represents a group of syndromes with different aetiological agents and because epidemiological studies lack uniform diagnostic criteria. There are few data available on morbidity and mortality; UK figures show eight deaths from occupational EAA, including farmer's lung, in 1998.

Pathogenesis and pathology

A wide variety of organic dusts can cause EAA, and the disease can be acute, subacute or chronic. A selection of antigens and sources of the disease is given in *Table 33*; the list is not comprehensive. The antigens may be fungal, bacterial, protozoal, animal or insect proteins, or low molecular weight chemical compounds. Commoner forms of EAA are generally provoked by thermophilic actinomycetes (spores of saprophytic fungi), fungi, and bird droppings.

Thermophilic actinomycetes are present in the atmosphere throughout the year. They most often produce disease when individuals are exposed to large numbers of particles, associated with abundant growth on decaying organic matter, enhanced by appropriate conditions of temperature and humidity. The spores can heavily contaminate a wide variety of vegetables, wood, sawdust, bark, water-reservoir humidifiers, and air-conditioning systems. Farmer's lung is associated with exposure to mouldy hay (a source of *Saccharopolyspora rectivirgula*, previously known as *Micropolyspora faeni*), but workers in many other different environments may be placed at risk.

The commonest form of avian-related EAA develops among pigeon fanciers, but similar symptoms can occur after exposure to budgerigars, parakeets, chickens, ducks, turkeys, and other small caged birds, such as finches and canaries (60). Avian antigens include droppings, feathers, and serum; a major antigen is thought to be bloom, which consists of keratin particles covered with IgA and is produced in large amounts by racing birds in peak condition.

The pathogenesis of EAA involves both humoral and cellular immune (T-cell mediated) responses. The time lapse between exposure and symptoms suggests a type III humoral immune reaction. EAA may be acute, subacute or chronic. Histologically, acute EAA is characterized by inflammation of the alveoli (alveolitis) and interstitium. There is lymphocyte infiltration with minimal fibrosis, and small noncaseating granulomas are present in two thirds of cases. The subacute form is characterized by bronchitis, and in chronic disease there is additional fibrosis.

Clinical features

Patients present with similar symptoms and clinical features regardless of the cause. Acute EAA is the form most often seen, and the easiest to characterize. Acute episodes usually follow sensitization; the intensity of the reaction is proportional to the amount of inhaled antigen and duration of exposure. Patients report acute systemic symptoms including fever, chills, chest tightness, breathlessness, and cough. Symptoms appear within hours of exposure and generally become manifest in the late afternoon or evening. Fever usually subsides by the morning but breathlessness may persist. With continued exposure to the provoking antigen, dyspnoea may become continuous.

Table 33 A selection of organic dusts causing extrinsic allergic alveolitis

Disease	Antigen	Source
Farmer's lung	*Saccharopolyspora rectivirgula*	Mouldy hay, grain or silage
Humidifier lung	*Thermoactinomyces vulgaris*, *T. sacchari*, *T. candidus*	Contaminated water reservoirs or forced air systems
Bagassosis	*Thermoactinomyces vulgaris*	Mouldy sugar cane
Malt worker's lung	*Aspergillus fumigatus, Aspergillus clavatus*	Mouldy barley
Pigeon-fancier's lung	Avian droppings, feathers, and serum	Pigeons, parakeets, budgerigars, chickens, turkeys
Cheese-washer's lung	*Penicillium casei, Aspergillus clavatus*	Mouldy cheese
Animal-handler's lung	Rats, gerbils	Urine, serum, pelts, proteins
Swimming pool worker's lung	Unknown	Aerolized endotoxin from pool-water sprays and fountains
Chemical worker's lung	Isocyanates, trimetallic anhydride	Polyurethane foams, spray paints, elastomers, special glues

The subacute form describes a more insidious onset of symptoms over weeks and months, and the chronic form is thought to be the sequel of acute or subacute disease. Patients with chronic disease frequently complain of a persistent productive cough. Inspiratory crackles are typically audible in acute EAA; finger clubbing may be present in chronic EAA.

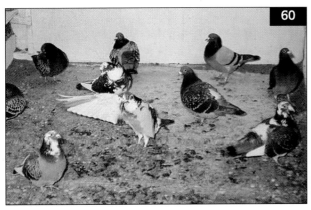

60 Pigeons are the cause of pigeon-fancier's lung, a common form of extrinsic allergic alveolitis. It results from sensitization to antigens in droppings, feathers, and serum. (Photo courtesy of Dr Gavin Boyd)

Table 34 Diffuse parenchymal lung disease associated with collagen vascular disease

❑ Rheumatoid arthritis
❑ Systemic sclerosis
❑ Mixed connective tissue disease
❑ Systemic lupus erythematosus
❑ Ankylosing spondylitis
❑ Behçet's disease
❑ Polymyositis and dermatomyositis
❑ Sjögren's syndrome

Table 35 Respiratory disease associated with rheumatoid arthritis

❑ Bronchiectasis
❑ Pleural disease (pleurisy, pleural effusion, empyema)
❑ Nodules
❑ Fibrosing alveolitis
❑ Cryptogenic organizing pneumonia
❑ Others (e.g. drug-induced lung disease, infection)

Investigations and diagnosis

Serum precipitating IgG antibodies against the causative antigen are usually detectable, but are also present in 10–50% of exposed, but asymptomatic, individuals. The presence of antigens thus merely indicates exposure and not disease. False negative results are also common. Chest radiographs and HRCT in early disease may show upper or lower zone patchy opacities. In chronic EAA there may be fibrosis indistinguishable from that seen in CFA. BAL usually shows a raised cell count with an increased proportion of lymphocytes and a predominance of CD8 T-cells. Transbronchial biopsy may provide adequate material to support a diagnosis, but open lung biopsy is not usually required in typical cases of acute EAA.

Management

Early diagnosis and avoidance of continued exposure to the antigen (where possible) are key. Continued antigen inhalation confers an adverse prognosis. Oral corticosteroids are recommended in acute, severe, and progressive disease. Steroids appear to hasten the resolution of acute EAA, but not to improve the long-term outcome.

DPLD ASSOCIATED WITH COLLAGEN VASCULAR DISEASE

Pulmonary involvement can be prominent in the systemic collagen vascular diseases, the two commonest of which are RA and systemic sclerosis. A more comprehensive list is provided in *Table 34*; details lie outside the scope of this book.

RHEUMATOID ARTHRITIS

RA is a symmetrical inflammatory polyarthropathy of unknown cause with a preponderance in females. It affects up to 100,000 patients in the UK and can cause a wide variety of pulmonary disorders (*Table 35*). Only DPLD is discussed here. Two distinct clinical syndromes may arise – fibrosing alveolitis and cryptogenic organizing pneumonia (COP – see *Table 38*, page 89). Fibrosing alveolitis associated with RA presents with a dry cough and progressive breathlessness. Bilateral basal crackles and finger clubbing are common. Pulmonary symptoms usually, but not always, follow the onset of arthritis.

Early in the course of the disease lung function tests may show little or no abnormality. In advanced disease the lung function abnormalities are identical to those seen in CFA. In early disease the chest radiograph shows bilateral, basal patchy alveolar infiltrates and, in more severe disease, this progresses to a reticular nodular pattern with honeycombing. HRCT features in late disease are similar to those of CFA, but in 20% of patients there is associated pleural disease.

BAL typically shows increased numbers of neutrophils and/or eosinophils. Lung biopsy may show fibrosis typical of CFA/UIP or a pattern of mixed inflammation and fibrosis. UK guidelines recommend similar management to that for CFA.

SYSTEMIC SCLEROSIS

Systemic sclerosis is a syndrome comprising inflammation and fibrosis of skin and internal organs. It mainly affects women and is associated with Raynaud's phenomenon and telangiectasia. Potential respiratory complications are listed in *Table 36*. DPLD is found especially in the presence of anti-Scl 70 antibodies. In contrast, patients with the anticentromere antibody (ACA) usually have limited disease and normal lung function. At post-mortem however, a degree of interstitial pulmonary fibrosis is almost universal in all patients dying of systemic sclerosis.

Patients may report breathlessness, and basal crackles may be present. The chest radiograph may show basal infiltrates or honeycombing. HRCT is more sensitive in detecting early lung involvement. Lung function tests show identical changes to those of CFA. BAL may show neutrophilia or eosinophilia. Surgical lung biopsy, if performed, reveals mixed inflammation and fibrosis.

Pulmonary fibrosis associated with systemic sclerosis has a better prognosis than CFA and lung function usually declines more slowly. Current UK guidelines recommend similar management to that for CFA, but cyclophosphamide is recommended as an alternative to azathioprine, combined with prednisolone.

SUMMARY OF DPLD ASSOCIATED WITH COLLAGEN VASCULAR DISEASE

❏ Pulmonary involvement can be prominent.
❏ The commonest causes are RA and systemic sclerosis.
❏ Fibrosing alveolitis in RA and systemic sclerosis has similar clinical features to that of CFA.
❏ The recommended treatment includes prednisolone and azathioprine.

DRUG- AND RADIATION-INDUCED DPLD

A wide variety of drugs can cause DPLD; some of the commoner ones are listed in *Table 37*. Patterns of disease are wide-ranging and include acute hypersensitivity pneumonitis, pneumonic infiltrates with eosinophilia, COP, and fibrosis.

Nitrofurantoin is one of the most frequent causes of drug-induced DPLD. Most commonly patients present with an acute hypersensitivity pneumonitis with fever, eosinophilia, myalgia, arthralgia, cough, and breathlessness after 1–3 weeks of treatment. Less common is a progressive chronic form of disease, with fibrosis following nitrofurantoin use for months or years.

Another frequent offender is amiodarone, which causes pulmonary toxicity in 5–10% of patients, especially at higher doses. In one third of cases an acute febrile pneumonitis occurs; the remaining two thirds

---

Table 36 Respiratory disease associated with systemic sclerosis

❏ Pulmonary arterial hypertension
❏ Chest wall restriction
❏ Fibrosing alveolitis
❏ Aspiration pneumonia (secondary to oesophageal dysmotility)

Table 37 A selection of drugs that may cause diffuse parenchymal lung disease (DPLD)

Drug	DPLD patterns
Amiodarone	Acute hypersensitivity pneumonitis; pulmonary fibrosis; COP; pulmonary nodules
Beta-blockers	Acute hypersensitivity pneumonitis; pneumonic infiltrates with eosinophilia; pulmonary fibrosis; COP
Bleomycin	Pneumonic infiltrates with eosinophilia; COP; pulmonary fibrosis; pulmonary nodules
Cyclophosphamide	Pneumonic infiltrates with eosinophilia; pulmonary fibrosis
Hydralazine	Cryptogenic organizing pneumonia
Methotrexate	Acute hypersensitivity pneumonitis; pneumonic infiltrates with eosinophilia
Nitrofurantoin	Acute hypersensitivity pneumonitis; pulmonary fibrosis

develop chronic fibrosing alveolitis. Rapidly progressive COP occasionally develops. Pulmonary abnormalities may persist or worsen after withdrawal of the drug. Corticosteroids may produce an improvement, but patients may relapse when they are stopped.

Illicit drugs can cause various respiratory complications; inhaled cocaine has been associated with several forms of DPLD, including pneumonic infiltrates with eosinophilia, and COP.

The pulmonary effects of radiation consist of acute radiation pneumonitis occurring 1–8 months after exposure, and chronic fibrosis occurring after 6–12 months. Symptoms may respond to oral corticosteroids, but patients may relapse when the dose is reduced.

SUMMARY OF DRUG-INDUCED DPLD
- ❑ Patterns of disease are varied.
- ❑ Amiodarone and nitrofurantoin are frequent causes.
- ❑ Not all conditions resolve on drug withdrawal.
- ❑ Corticosteroids are indicated in some circumstances.

RARE DPLDS
Table 38 lists some of the more unusual forms of DPLD, with an outline of their particular characteristics. The student is referred to the 'recommended reading' section at the end of this chapter for specialist reviews.

Table 38 Some unusual forms of diffuse parenchymal lung disease with distinguishing features

Condition	Distinguishing features
Alveolar proteinosis	Unknown aetiology. Alveoli filled with lipoproteinaceous material derived from surfactant components. 'Crazy paving' pattern on HRCT. Diagnosed on BAL. Responds well to whole lung lavage
Amyloidosis	Extracellular accumulation of fibrillary proteins staining positively with Congo red and exhibiting green birefringence under polarized light. May cause parenchymal nodules or diffuse reticulonodular infiltrates on HRCT
Cryptogenic organizing pneumonia (COP)	Symptoms often mimic pneumonia, with persistent nonproductive cough, breathlessness, fever, malaise, fatigue, and weight loss. CXR shows bilateral, diffuse alveolar opacities, often recurrent and migratory. Histology shows organizing pneumonia (proliferation of granulation tissue within small airways). Two thirds of patients recover with oral corticosteroids
Goodpasture's syndrome (antibasement membrane antibody disease)	Characterized by glomerulonephritis with or without pulmonary haemorrhage
Lymphangioleiomyomatosis (LAM)	Affects pre-menopausal females. Proliferation of smooth muscle cells (probably hormone-dependent) leads to airflow obstruction and cysts on HRCT. Causes dyspnoea, haemoptysis, recurrent pneumothoraces, and chylous effusions
Langerhans cell histiocytosis (histiocytosis X)	Adult disease predominantly affects young cigarette smokers. Affected tissues are infiltrated by Langerhan's cells. Cysts and nodules on HRCT
Neurofibromatosis	Autosomal dominant. Results from proliferation of the neural crest and can affect any organ. Type I (von Recklinghausen's disease) is the commonest form. 20% of these develop lower zone reticulonodular infiltrates and bullous changes in the upper zones
Pulmonary eosinophilia (eosinophilic pneumonia)	Typically causes infiltrates on CXR and peripheral blood eosinophilia. May result from fungal exposure (especially allergic bronchopulmonary aspergillosis), drugs, parasite infections, or arise with no obvious cause
Pulmonary vasculitis	Wegner's granulomatosis, Churg–Strauss syndrome, and microscopic polyangiitis are the three commonest forms
Tuberous sclerosis	Autosomal dominant condition with equal sex incidence and variable expression. Classic triad consists of dermal angiofibroma (adenoma sebaceum), epilepsy, and mental retardation. HRCT features may be cystic and reticular. Histological changes are identical to those of LAM

HRCT, high-resolution computed tomography; BAL, bronchoalveolar lavage; CXR, chest radiograph

SUMMARY OF DIFFUSE PARENCHYMAL LUNG DISEASE

- ❏ DPLD denotes around 200 conditions affecting the lung parenchyma.
- ❏ Commoner conditions include sarcoidosis, cryptogenic fibrosing alveolitis (CFA), occupational and recreational DPLD, DPLD associated with collagen vascular disease, and drug-induced DPLD.
- ❏ In many cases the aetiology is unclear.
- ❏ Lung biopsy may be required to establish a precise diagnosis.
- ❏ Prognosis may be poor (e.g. CFA).
- ❏ Specific treatment options include removal of the patient from exposure to the offending agent (if known), corticosteroids with or without additional immunosuppressants, and lung transplantation.
- ❏ Supportive management includes treating hypoxia and any associated pulmonary hypertension.

RECOMMENDED READING

The Diffuse Parenchymal Lung Disease Group, British Thoracic Society, Standards of Care Committee. The diagnosis, assessment and treatment of diffuse parenchymal lung disease in adults. *Thorax* 1999;**54**(Suppl. 1):1–30.

American Thoracic Society statement on sarcoidosis *American Journal of Respiratory Critical Care Medicine* 1999;**160**: 736–55

www.pneumotox.com; this website collates reports of drug-induced lung disease and is a useful on-line reference. Not all these reports fall into the category of DPLD.

Chapter 9 Pleural diseases

INTRODUCTION

The pleura is a serous membrane that covers the lung, the mediastinum, the diaphragm, and the rib cage. It is comprised of a visceral layer that covers the lung parenchyma and a parietal layer that lines the inside of the thoracic cavity. A thin film of fluid, pleural fluid, acts as a lubricant to enable normal lung movement during respiration. The area occupied by this thin layer of fluid is the pleural space. Pleural fluid normally originates from within the capillaries in the parietal pleura and is cleared by lymphatics in the same way. The normal volume of pleural fluid in a healthy individual is 1–5 ml although the turnover of pleural fluid is thought to be between 1 and 2 l/day. The hydrostatic gradient in the capillaries in the parietal pleura favours an efflux of fluid into the pleural space. Pressure in the capillaries in the visceral pleura is lower in keeping with that of the pulmonary capillaries. This lower pressure favours resorption of fluid from the visceral surface.

PLEURAL EFFUSIONS

Pleural effusions develop when there is a discrepancy between the formation of and resorption of the pleural fluid. This leads to an excessive accumulation of fluid – which can comprise a variety of liquids including blood, pus, and chyle – in the pleural space. There may be various reasons for this imbalance:
- ❏ Increased microvascular hydrostatic pressure.
- ❏ Reduced vascular oncotic pressure.
- ❏ Impaired lymphatic drainage.
- ❏ Increased microvascular permeability.
- ❏ Reduced pleural space pressure.
- ❏ Fluid transfer from peritoneum/abnormal sites of entry.

Disease processes that may cause the above states are shown in *Table 39*.

CLINICAL FEATURES

The cardinal features of pleural disease are pleuritic pain, cough, and breathlessness. Pleuritic pain is a sharp pain felt most intensely with deep inspiration, coughing, and sneezing. It suggests inflammation of the underlying parietal pleura, as the visceral pleura does not have pain fibres. If the pleura itself is not inflamed some patients may just experience a dull, dragging feeling or aching rather than pain. Many patients experience a dry cough. This may be related either to the pleural inflammation or the compression of segmental bronchi stimulating the cough reflex. The other common symptom of a pleural effusion is breathlessness, but this depends on the size of the effusion. A large effusion compresses the lung and reduces all sub-divisions of lung segment volumes. Diaphragmatic function may also be compromised and this may exacerbate breathlessness.

Abnormal physical signs may be absent if the effusion is small. If a larger effusion is present there may be reduced chest wall expansion on the side of the effusion with displacement of the trachea away from the effusion. Palpation of the chest wall can be

Table 39 Mechanism for pleural fluid accumulation	
Mechanism	**Cause**
Increased microvascular hydrostatic pressure	Raised venous pressure (heart failure, constrictive pericarditis)
Reduced vascular oncotic pressure	Hypoalbuminaemia (cirrhosis, nephrotic syndrome)
Impaired lymphatic drainage	Lymphatic obstruction (mediastinal lymph nodes)
Increased microvascular permeability	Infection/inflammation (pneumonia, collagen diseases)
Reduced pleural space pressure	Atelectasis (collapsed lobe/lung)
Fluid transfer from peritoneum/abnormal sites of entry	Diaphragmatic weakness Ascites Peritoneal dialysis

diagnostic. The percussion note is stony–dull, and tactile vocal fremitus is absent or attenuated. Tactile vocal fremitus or vocal resonance is a very reliable way for ascertaining the top of the effusion, where the amount of fluid is at its least. Auscultation reveals absent or diminished breath sounds over the effusion. At the superior border of the fluid, breath sounds may be bronchial in nature.

INVESTIGATIONS AND DIAGNOSIS

Pleural fluid accumulates in the most dependent part of the thoracic cavity, as the lung is less dense than the pleural fluid. Firstly the fluid rests between the inferior surface of the lung and the diaphragm. A PA chest radiograph is the best way to visualize an effusion, although it adds little to understanding its aetiology. 300 ml of fluid will result in blunting of the costophrenic angle (61). In uncomplicated large effusions the trachea and mediastinum are shifted away from the effusion (62). If this is not seen it may indicate the presence of an underlying lobar collapse, suggestive of a primary bronchogenic tumour with an associated effusion (63). Pleural effusions can occur bilaterally. This is more common with transudates, when the right effusion is often greater than the left.

An ultrasound scan is useful to locate a small effusion and can detect areas of loculation (pleural strands and debris) which may be indicative of an empyema.

CT can demonstrate much smaller effusions than a plain chest radiograph and can also estimate the thickness of the pleura and assess the underlying lung. It is, however, not part of the routine investigation of an effusion.

Diagnosis is by pleural aspiration. An excess of fluid can be detected on a plain chest radiograph when there is more than 300 ml and clinically detected with more than 500 ml. The patient should be sitting in a comfortable upright position. The fluid level should be percussed/auscultated and an area marked one intercostal space below the top of the effusion. Ultrasonography can be used in small effusions to mark the best area from which to withdraw fluid. The process must be performed under strict aseptic technique. The skin and subcutaneous tissues are infiltrated with 1 or 2% lignocaine. As the intercostal

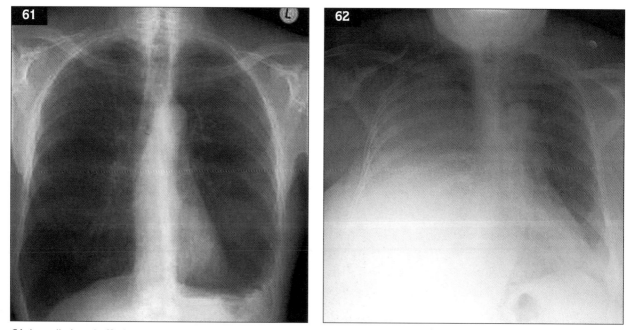

61 A small pleural effusion with blunting of the costophrenic angle

62 A large pleural effusion with mediastinal shift

bundle (intercostal vein, artery, and nerve) lies beneath the rib the needle should be carefully inserted along the superior surface of the rib. For diagnostic purposes between 50 and 100 ml should be removed using a 30 ml syringe and green (21G) cannula. *Table 40* shows the tests that should be requested when investigating an undiagnosed pleural effusion.

For therapeutic aspiration to relieve breathlessness a small cannula should be inserted to minimize damage to the underlying lung and maximize ease of fluid withdrawal.

EXAMINATION OF PLEURAL FLUID

Appearance

The gross appearance of pleural fluid (colour, viscosity, and turbidity) can be very informative and should be recorded in the notes. Most effusions are clear, straw coloured, non-viscid, and odourless. A red/pink effusion is suggestive of blood and this is likely to indicate malignancy, trauma or a pulmonary infarction. If the fluid is very dark red a haematocrit should be performed. If this is > 50% of the peripheral haematocrit a haemothorax (see page 95)

is present that will require tube drainage. Turbid fluid suggests increased cellular content and points towards infection. Milky white turbid fluid suggests the presence of chyle.

Biochemistry

In clinical practice the majority of effusions are either transudates or exudates, which can be distiguished by simple biochemical analysis of the pleural fluid. Effusions with protein levels < 30 g/l are transudates and those with levels > 30 g/l are classified as exudates. There can be significant overlap within these levels and to improve sensitivity and specificity the lactate dehydrogenase (LDH) level should also be measured. The levels of protein and LDH in the effusion can then be compared to the serum levels to improve diagnostic certainty as shown below.

To define an exudate:
❏ Pleural fluid protein:serum protein ratio > 0.5.
❏ Pleural fluid LDH:serum LDH ratio > 0.6.
❏ Pleural fluid LDH > 200 IU.

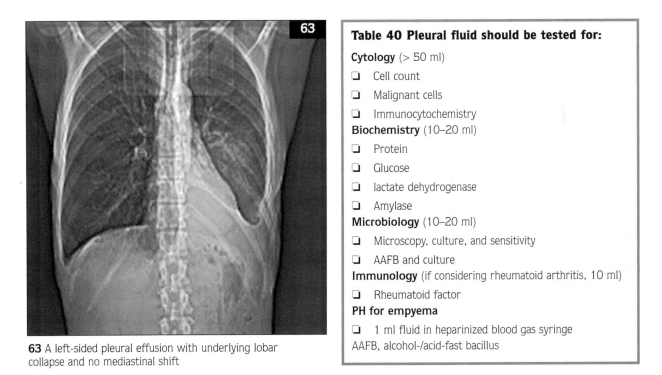

63 A left-sided pleural effusion with underlying lobar collapse and no mediastinal shift

Table 40 Pleural fluid should be tested for:

Cytology (> 50 ml)
❏ Cell count
❏ Malignant cells
❏ Immunocytochemistry
Biochemistry (10–20 ml)
❏ Protein
❏ Glucose
❏ lactate dehydrogenase
❏ Amylase
Microbiology (10–20 ml)
❏ Microscopy, culture, and sensitivity
❏ AAFB and culture
Immunology (if considering rheumatoid arthritis, 10 ml)
❏ Rheumatoid factor
PH for empyema
❏ 1 ml fluid in heparinized blood gas syringe
AAFB, alcohol-/acid-fast bacillus

Common causes of transudates and exudates are shown in *Table 41*.

Glucose is not routinely measured and the sample has to be sent in a special bottle. A low pleural fluid glucose level compared to the serum glucose can suggest RA or severe infection. If pancreatitis is the cause of the effusion, pleural fluid amylase will be high.

Cell count
Cell counts can be obtained in two ways: either by sending some fluid to haematology for a coulter count (warn haematology that it is pleural fluid) or via cytology. It is important to know the breakdown of leucocytes within the fluid (*Table 42*).

Cytology
At least 50 ml of fluid must be sent to cytology for an adequate assessment. It can be difficult to differentiate between an adenocarcinoma and a mesothelioma so immunohistochemistry is required. When sending a sample to cytology it is imperative to put as much relevant information as possible on the request form to aid the cytopathologist.

Microbiology
Fluid should always be sent for a Gram stain and culture including TB culture. If an anaerobic infection is suspected (i.e. an empyema) the fluid should be taken to the microbiology laboratory as quickly as possible and anaerobic cultures requested.

Pleural biopsy
If the initial aspirate is nondiagnostic a pleural biopsy may be indicated. This can be done in one of three ways: 'blind' on the ward with an Abram's needle; under CT guidance with a cutting needle; in theatre under a general anaesthetic using key hole (video-assisted) surgery (thoracoscopy).

Indications for the use of an Abram's needle include a high suspicion of TB. In the diagnosis of TB the culture of biopsy fragments increases the pick-up from 25% for fluid culture alone up to 80% if the biopsies are taken by specialist respiratory teams. The presence of caseating granulomas at histology is also diagnostic. Abram's biopsy is also indicated if the suspicion of malignancy is high and the patient's prognosis is poor (i.e. life expectancy < 3 months) because it avoids more invasive diagnostic procedures.

If there is evidence of localized pleural thickening or a mass then CT can be used to guide a cutting needle to the right area.

For patients with undiagnosed effusions, particularly if suspicious for malignancy, the treatment of choice is video-assisted thoracoscopic surgery (VATS). This entails a general anaesthetic so the patient has to be reasonably fit, with a life expectancy of > 3 months. During VATS the pleura is inspected and any abnormal areas directly sampled. If there is obvious malignancy all the fluid can be drained in theatre and talc applied to the pleural surface to prevent the effusion from recurring. Thus a diagnostic and therapeutic procedure will have occurred simultaneously.

Table 41 Differential diagnosis of pleural effusion

Transudates	Infectious	Gastrointestinal disease
❏ Congestive cardiac failure	❏ Infectious	❏ Gastrointestinal disease
❏ Cirrhosis	Bacterial	Sub-phrenic collection
❏ Nephrotic syndrome	Tuberculosis	Pancreatitis
❏ Hypoalbuminaemia	Atypical (rare)	Post abdominal surgery
❏ Peritoneal dialysis	Fungal	Oesophageal rupture
❏ Myxoedema	❏ Pulmonary emboli	❏ Heart disease
❏ Pulmonary emboli	❏ Collagen vascular disease	Post coronary artery bypass
❏ Sarcoidosis	Rheumatoid arthritis	graft
Exudates	SLE	Dressler's syndrome
❏ Malignancy	Sjögren's syndrome	❏ Obstetrical & gynaecological
Metastatic disease	ANCA associated diseases	Post partum
Mesothelioma		Ovarian hyperstimulation
Lymphoma		syndrome
		Meigs's syndrome

ANCA, antineutrophil cytoplasmic antibody; SLE, systemic lupus erythematosus

Table 42 Cell counts to help in the differential diagnosis of pleural effusions

Cell type	Count	Disease process
Red blood cell	>100,000/mm^3	Trauma Malignancy Pulmonary embolism
	Haematocrit >50% serum	Haemothorax
White blood cells	>10,000/mm^3	Pyogenic infection
Neutrophils	>50%	Pyogenic infection
Lymphocytes	>90%	Tuberculosis Lymphoma Malignancy
Eosinophils	>10%	Repeated aspirations Lymphoma

TREATMENT

Treatment must involve treating the underlying condition; an empyema requires urgent drainage and is dealt with separately later.

Malignant pleural effusions can be difficult to treat as the effusion often re-accumulates quickly. The commonest malignant effusions are due to lung cancer or breast cancer. It is unusual for the effusion to subside following chemotherapy so specific measures have to be undertaken. If the patient has a good quality of life and good performance score (see Chapter 5, page 45) a VATS procedure and a talc pleurodesis could be undertaken. If the patient is not fit enough for a general anaesthetic a medical pleurodesis can be attempted. The effusion is first drained to dryness with a small-bore catheter or intercostal drain. A sclerosing agent is then instilled into the pleural cavity. This can be very painful for the patient so lidocaine may be instilled first. Tetracycline used to be the agent of choice for medical pleurodesis, but owing to limited supplies, it is now more common to use sterile talc. This is made into a sterile slurry at the bedside and instilled into the drain. The drain is clamped and the patient asked to rotate to allow the slurry to mix throughout the pleural space. The remaining slurry is then allowed to drain out (often on suction). Medical pleurodesis is successful in about 60% of cases (75% for talc, 50% for tetracycline).

Empyema

Empyema is the presence of a purulent pleural effusion where there is an excess of white cells and inflammatory cells, suggestive of active infection. Empyema can follow a simple pneumonia or can occur in the presence of a lung abscess or bronchiectasis. A simple exudative effusion can become an empyema if nonsterile techniques are used while performing an aspiration. Empyema can occur with septicaemia, after medical thoracocentesis, after thoracic surgery or following a penetrating chest wound. Tuberculous empyema is rare nowadays in the UK.

The patient will have the clinical signs of an effusion but may have a swinging pyrexia and an acute serological inflammatory response. The chest radiograph may show a simple effusion or a loculated effusion. A diagnostic aspirate must be taken as soon as possible. An empyema is present if the fluid is turbid or purulent. It will be an acidic exudate (pH < 7.2 as measured in a blood gas analyser) with a very high LDH (often > 1,000 IU) and low glucose. A Gram stain may reveal the organism responsible and immediate culture is required to grow any anaerobes.

Treatment involves immediate intercostal tube drainage and commencement of appropriate antibiotics. The initial choice of antibiotics is often made without culture results, so must include cover for streptococci as well as Gram-negative organisms and anaerobes. The usual first-line choice is intravenous cefuroxime with metronidazole. Antibiotics alone are not enough to clear an empyema. If the pus is not adequately draining through the intercostal drain an intrapleural thrombolytic agent can be introduced to break down loculations. This is currently the subject of a MRC trial to determine if the use of streptokinase prevents the need for surgical drainage. If an empyema does not drain the patient may require formal thoracotomy with clearance of the pleural space and decortication. Antibiotics should be continued for 2–3 weeks post surgery and for up to 6 weeks if surgery is not used.

HAEMOTHORAX

A true haemothorax is diagnosed if the level of haematocrit in the pleural fluid is > 50% of that in the serum. The commonest causes are a penetrating chest injury or nonpenetrating deceleration injuries. Occasionally haemothoraces can be iatrogenic from central venous lines or the insertion of pacemakers. Rare causes include rupture of the ascending aorta and excess anticoagulation.

The treatment of choice is to insert a very large bore chest drain (> 28 French) to allow drainage of any clots. The presence of continued bleeding can be monitored via such drainage; continued bleeding may require a thoracotomy.

CHYLOTHORAX

This is due to the accumulation of lymph in the pleural space. Absorbed fat is transported as chylomicrons into the bloodstream via the thoracic duct. The thoracic duct can be injured during mobilization in oesophageal and aortic surgery. Penetrating trauma and deceleration injuries can also tear the thoracic duct. Malignant infiltration of the duct with lymphomas is the commonest malignant cause of a chylothorax.

Diagnosis is by the aspiration of milky white fluid from the pleural space. Unlike an empyema there are few white cells and a smear shows cholesterol crystals. Insertion of a chest drain will remove the chyle but reaccumulation will occur quickly. To reduce the flow of chyle the patient must be fed with a medium-chain fatty acid diet only. If the thoracic duct is leaking this needs to be surgically repaired. Malignant infiltration can be palliated with radiotherapy.

PNEUMOTHORAX

A pneumothorax occurs when air is introduced into the pleural space. This may be spontaneous or occur following trauma. Spontaneous (primary) pneumo-thoraces occur mostly in tall thin young (aesthenic) men, where sub-pleural blebs in the lung apices can rupture into the pleural space. The incidence is about 10 per 100,000 population and the male:female ratio is 4:1. The peak age is mid-20s and primary sponta-neous pneumothoraces rarely occur after the age of 40. Pneumothoraces are likely to recur with a recurrence rate of over 40% within 2 years.

Secondary pneumothoraces occur when the underlying lung is diseased, for example secondary to COPD or asthma.

Pneumothoraces can be caused iatrogenically when central venous lines are being inserted, when transbronchial biopsies are being performed, or during fine needle aspiration biopsy of solitary pulmonary masses. Patients should always be warned of this possibility.

Spontaneous pneumothorax often presents with pleuritic pain and breathlessness. The pain is of sudden onset and unilateral to the side of the pneumothorax. The degree of breathlessness depends on the size of the pneumothorax.

Clinical signs vary according to the size of the pneumothorax. There may be few signs with a small air leak. As the pneumothorax enlarges the patient may become more tachypnoeic, tachycardic, and hypoxic. There may be evidence of mediastinal shift. Percussion will be resonant on the affected side with absent breath sounds. If the pneumothorax is under tension (64) it is an emergency, as the patient may become hypotensive and collapse (*Table 43*).

If the patient is not in a collapsed state, confirmation of the pneumothorax is best made with a plain chest radiograph. Expiratory images are not routinely required but they or a lateral image may be helpful if a small pneumothorax is suspected. If a tension pneumothorax is suspected clinically, air must

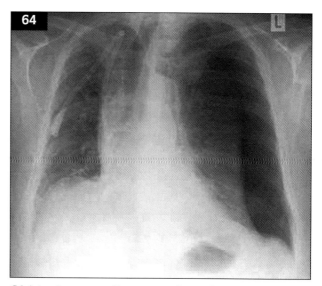

64 A tension pneumothorax; note the mediastinal and tracheal shift

Table 43 Tension pneumothorax

Signs
- ❏ Respiratory distress
- ❏ Tachypneoic
- ❏ Tachycardic
- ❏ Hypotensive
- ❏ Cardiac arrest

On examination – this is a clinical diagnosis
- ❏ No air entry on one side
- ❏ Mediastinum shifted to other side
- ❏ Distended neck veins

Treatment
- ❏ Attempt resuscitation before obtaining a chest radiograph
- ❏ Attach a 20 ml syringe containing 5 ml saline to a 16 G cannula
- ❏ Insert cannula into 2nd intercostal space, midclavicular line on suspected side
- ❏ Remove plunger
- ❏ Allow air to bubble through saline
- ❏ Obtain a chest radiograph
- ❏ Set up for a formal intercostal drain

be aspirated urgently. In patients with severe bullous emphysema, a CT scan can sometimes aid the placement of an intercostal drain to avoid placing the drain into a bulla.

The management of different sized pneumo-thoraces is outlined in figure 65. Aspiration of air is safe and simple and is described in *Table 44*.

For the safe placement of an intercostal tube drain it is recommended that the drain be placed within the safe triangle to minimize the risk to other structures (66). Intercostal tube drainage is discussed further in *Table 45*.

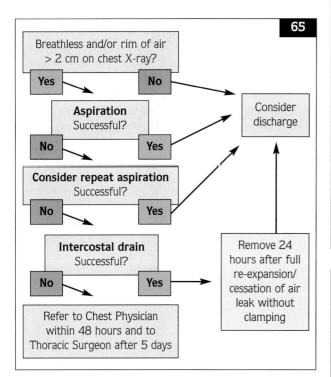

65 The management of a primary pneumothorax

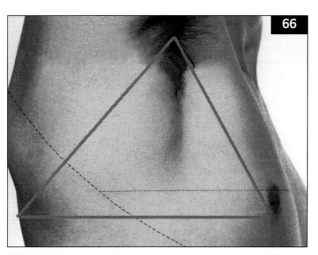

66 The 'safe triangle' for the insertion of an intercostal drain

---

Table 44 Aspiration of a pneumothorax

Equipment
- ❑ Full sterile kit (gown, gloves, dressing pack, and towels)
- ❑ 10 ml 1% lignocaine
- ❑ Three-way tap

Selection of 19–23 G needles
- ❑ 10 ml and 50 ml syringes
- ❑ 16 G plastic cannula

Technique
- ❑ Sterilize the anterior chest wall
- ❑ Identify the site for drainage as the 2nd anterior intercostal space in the midclavicular line
- ❑ Anaesthetize the skin and deep tissues to the pleura
- ❑ Place the catheter into the above space
- ❑ Remove the inner needle and attach three-way tap
- ❑ Using 50 ml syringe aspirate air until no more can be aspirated or resistance is felt

---

Table 45 Use of intercostal drains

Type of intercostal drain
- ❑ For most pleural effusions and pneumothoraces small-bore chest drains (12 to 14 F) can be used
- ❑ Small-bore chest drains usually come pre-packed with all the equipment needed, including guide wire and dilator
- ❑ 14 F drains can be used for the management of an empyema
- ❑ Haemothoraces require large-bore (> 26 F) chest drains

Position of drain
- ❑ For effusions the drain should be one intercostal space below the level of the effusion, with the tip directed downwards
- ❑ For pneumothoraces drains should be placed in the 'safe triangle' with the tip angled towards the apex

Insertion of intercostal drains
- ❑ All drains must be placed under full sterile procedure
- ❑ Local anaesthetic is usually all that is required. If placing large-bore drains systemic analgesia with pethidine may be required pre-procedure
- ❑ 14 F drains are placed using a Seldinger guidewire technique
- ❑ Large-bore drains must be placed using blunt dissection into the pleural space; the trocar should never be used to enter the pleural space

If left alone in an asymptomatic patient air will be spontaneously resorbed from the pleural space at 1.25% of the total hemithorax per day. Therefore, a pneumothorax occupying 15% of the hemithorax would take 12 days to be completely absorbed. Even though recurrent spontaneous pneumothoraces may resolve spontaneously, there may be a case for surgical intervention to prevent recurrences, especially after a second pneumothorax on the same side. A lower threshold for early intervention, even after one pneumo-thorax, may be appropriate in those who fly frequently or in those living in areas far from medical care.

If the pneumothorax is still present after 3–4 days, or there is constant bubbling, it suggests that there is a persistent air leak or a bronchopleural fistula. The underwater drain can be placed on low-pressure suction (2–5 kPa or 15–20 cmH$_2$O). For this a special low-pressure suction unit has to be used, as most wall -based suction units are high pressure (> 20 kPa) and can cause significant barotrauma if attached by mistake. If the air leak does not seal under suction the patient is likely to require a thoracotomy. This will most probably involve a VATS procedure. Any apical blebs can be localized and removed using a staple gun. To prevent future pneumothoraces the surgeon will perform either a pleurectomy or a talc pleurodesis. Figure **67** identifies the management strategy of a secondary pneumothorax.

PLEURAL PLAQUES

Pleural plaques associated with exposure to asbestos are common but not actual tumours. There is no evidence that pleural plaques transform into pleural tumours.

PLEURAL TUMOURS

Primary pleural tumours are rare.

BENIGN TUMOURS

Pleural fibrous mesothelioma (pleural fibroma, solitary fibrous tumour) are the most common benign tumours, but even so they are very uncommon. Most patients have no previous exposure to asbestos. Most of these tumours arise from the visceral pleura and are characterized by sheets of benign spindle cells with no malignant differentiation. The median age of presentation is 60 years. Most patients are asympto-matic and present because of an abnormal routine chest radiograph. In the remaining patients, most present with chest pain and breathlessness. Patients may be clubbed or have HOA, and rarely have hypoglycaemia.

On a chest radiograph the mass may appear as a peripheral tumour, in the form of a mediastinal mass. CT further characterizes the tumour as a solitary inhomogeneous mass (**68**). Diagnosis can be made by a tru-cut biopsy or at thoracotomy. Surgical excision is the treatment of choice and is curative in 90% of cases.

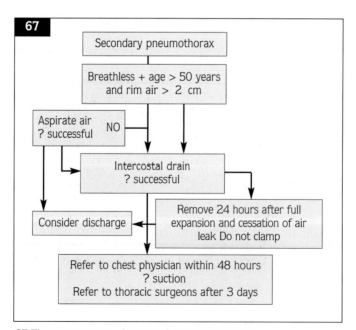

67 The management of a secondary pneumothorax

MALIGNANT MESOTHELIOMA

Malignant mesothelioma is thought to arise from the mesothelial cells that line the pleural cavity. It was recognized in the 1960s that there is a strong link between the development of mesothelioma and exposure to asbestos, though there is a latent period of 20–40 years before the disease may become manifest. The risk for developing mesothelioma relates to the type of asbestos and length of exposure.

Asbestos is a fibrous silicate of various chemical types. Fibres with the greatest length to diameter ratio are the most carcinogenic as they take such a long time to be cleared from the lungs. Chrysotile (white asbestos) is the most common asbestos fibre and has a low risk of malignancy – unless there is very prolonged exposure – as the fibres are cleared from the lungs in a few weeks. Crocidolite (blue asbestos) is much more carcinogenic, even with short exposure times, and can take decades to be cleared from the lungs. Although the risk of asbestos-related malignancy is now known the incidence of mesothelioma will continue to rise until 2020.

In its earliest stages mesothelioma appears as white nodules or flakes on the parietal pleura. Ten percent of mesothelioma can arise in the peritoneum. As the tumour progresses the pleural surface thickens and the tumour expands in all directions. This tumour layer then encases the lungs and contracts the hemithorax. In advanced cases the heart and mediastinal structures may be involved.

The age of presentation is between 50 and 70 years of age and there is a preponderance of the disease in males owing to exposure at work. Most patients present with insidious onset breathlessness and chest pain. The pain is often referred to the shoulder and upper abdomen because of involvement of the diaphragm. As the disease progresses patients lose weight and become more breathless. There may be fevers and night sweats.

On examination clubbing is rare. The only clinical findings will be related to a pleural effusion or restricted hemithorax movement in late disease. A chest radiograph will show a pleural effusion in 90% of cases. Pleural plaques may be visible in the other hemithorax. In advanced disease there may be obvious volume loss on the side of the mesothelioma. Further staging is required with a CT scan to assess the extent of pleural thickening and any disease extension into the mediastinum, chest wall or abdomen (**69**).

Pleural fluid must be sent for cytological analysis. Immunocytochemistry on pleural fluid has the highest diagnostic value for mesothelioma and can differentiate the tumour from an adenocarcinoma. If pleural fluid cytology is negative a CT-guided biopsy or open biopsy should be sought. At surgery, it is possible to

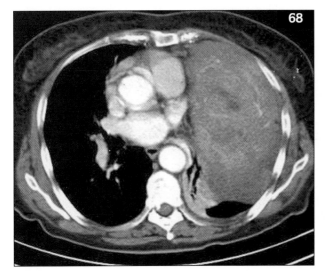

68 A pleural fibroma

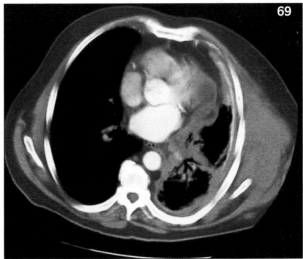

69 Malignant mesothelioma encasing the left lung and extending into the mediastinum and chest wall

stage the mesothelioma further. If the disease is advanced a talc pleurodesis can be performed to minimize fluid recurrence. In very limited disease (small volume parietal pleural disease with no visceral extension or lymph node involvement) radical surgery can occasionally be attempted and is the subject of a current multi-centre trial.

There is no curative treatment for mesothelioma apart from a few selected cases (as above) who undergo extrapleural pneumonectomy, the mortality from which is 25%. All patients must have palliative radiotherapy to any surgical or biopsy entrance sites to prevent disease tracking into the skin. Palliative radiotherapy can control pain for a period of time.

Chemotherapy is an area still under investigation for mesothelioma. There are reports of good symptom control and some evidence of disease regression. The most important aspect of care is good palliative care and symptom control. There should be early involvement of the palliative care team and pain control team. Median survival is 18 months.

Patients should be advised of their entitlement to government compensation and be advised to seek legal advice regarding damages from their employers. In the UK advice may be sought from The Occupational and Environmental Diseases Association, Mitre House, 66 Abbey Road, Bush Hill Park, Enfield, Middlesex EN1 2QH.

CASE STUDIES

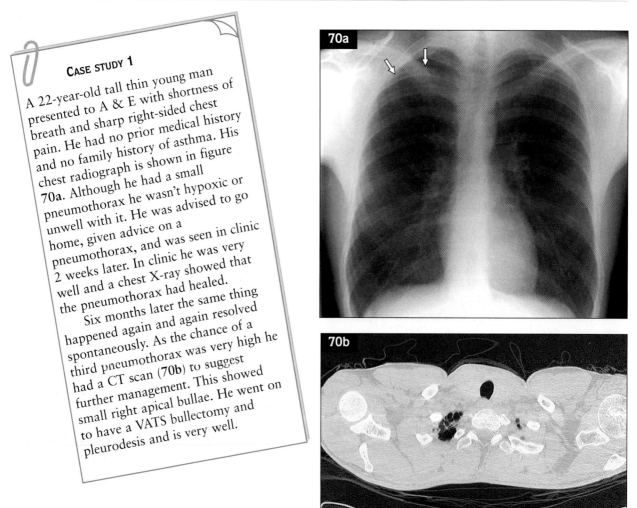

CASE STUDY 1

A 22-year-old tall thin young man presented to A & E with shortness of breath and sharp right-sided chest pain. He had no prior medical history and no family history of asthma. His chest radiograph is shown in figure 70a. Although he had a small pneumothorax he wasn't hypoxic or unwell with it. He was advised to go home, given advice on a pneumothorax, and was seen in clinic 2 weeks later. In clinic he was very well and a chest X-ray showed that the pneumothorax had healed.

Six months later the same thing happened again and again resolved spontaneously. As the chance of a third pneumothorax was very high he had a CT scan (70b) to suggest further management. This showed small right apical bullae. He went on to have a VATS bullectomy and pleurodesis and is very well.

70 (a) A small pneumothorax (arrowed); (b) CT thorax showing apical bullae in the same person as (a)

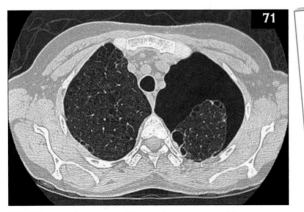

71 CT scan of a pneumothorax in a woman with bullous emphysema

CASE STUDY 2

A 55-year-old woman who was a lifelong smoker came in to A & E very breathless. She was hypoxic and had low oxygen saturations. Her chest radiograph showed a large pneumothorax. Aspiration of air was unsuccessful so a small intercostal drain was inserted. Despite a well positioned drain and the use of suction the lung did not expand. A CT scan (71) showed a partly deflated left lung and emphysema. She went on to have a VATS talc pleurodesis to good effect. She has successfully given up smoking.

CASE STUDY 3

A 75-year-old woman with vasculitis and renal failure was referred for further investigation of a left upper lobe cavity. She was a lifelong smoker and was on immunosuppresive treatment for her vasculitis. The differential diagnosis was a cavitating squamous cell carcinoma, TB or a fungal cavity.

She proceeded to have a CT-guided lung biopsy, which was performed without complication. A post biopsy chest radiograph showed no pneumothorax so she was sent back to the ward. 5 hours later the Senior House Officer (SHO) was called as she was very breathless, sweaty, tachycardic, and hypotensive. The SHO heard no air entry on the left side and the trachea was shifted to the right. The SHO immediately inserted a 16 G cannula into the left thoracic cavity with immediate improvement. A drain was subsequently inserted.

SUMMARY

- ❑ The commonest causes of a pleural effusion are heart failure, pneumonia, and lung cancer.
- ❑ It is imperative to work out whether the effusion is an exudate or a transudate.
- ❑ Pus in the pleural space indicates an empyema and is a medical/surgical emergency.
- ❑ A tension pneumothorax is a medical emergency.
- ❑ Most pleural effusions and pneumothoraces can be treated with small-bore catheters which cause minimal trauma for the patient.
- ❑ Understand the location of the safe triangle for the insertion of drains for pneumothoraces.

Chapter 10 Infections of the respiratory tract

INTRODUCTION

The respiratory tract is in direct communication with the external environment and offers an accessible portal for infections. Infections of the respiratory tract, upper and lower, are therefore very common and cause much morbidity, leading to around 10% of all consultations in general practice. The vast majority of these infections follow a benign course and patients make an uneventful recovery, while a small proportion, particularly among children, the elderly, and the immunocompromised, run the risk of a poorer outcome. The various infections of the respiratory tract are listed in the schematic diagram below (**72**).

UPPER RESPIRATORY TRACT INFECTIONS

These are extremely common and are mostly caused by viruses. They do not require any specific therapy and antibiotics do not have a role to play in their management, except in the specific circumstances mentioned below. Rest, adequate hydration, and analgesics for the systemic symptoms (headache, body aches) are the mainstay of treatment.

INFLUENZA

Of the three types of influenza virus (A, B and C), type A is the most and type C the least pathogenic. Minor ('antigenic drift') and major ('antigenic shift') alterations in the genotype result in increasing infectivity, with antigenic shifts sometimes leading to worldwide epidemics. The disease is highly infectious and typically presents with acute onset fever, cough, headache, sore throat, nasal congestion, and myalgia. Symptoms of pneumonia (see below) may follow, either as a manifestation of the viral illness or owing to a secondary bacterial infection caused by *Staphylococcus*, *Pneumococcus* or *Haemophilus* spp.. Specific antiviral treatment is not usually required but the antiviral agent zanamivir is available, although not widely recommended, for use early in the disease to decrease its duration and severity.

Annual vaccination against influenza is recommended in the elderly and in patients with COPD, other chronic respiratory disorders, heart failure, renal failure, and diabetes. The vaccine, which is based on the serotypes considered most likely to cause infection that year, is around 70% effective and, even if not effective in preventing infection, often lessens the severity of the illness.

SINUSITIS

Sinusitis results from infection of the maxillary and, less commonly, the frontal paranasal sinuses by bacteria and viruses (**72**). The symptoms include headaches, facial pain, fever, cough (sometimes nocturnal due to a 'postnasal drip') productive of purulent sputum. Sinusitis may occasionally be associated with primary ciliary dyskinesia causing bronchiectasis, situs inversus (Kartagener's syndrome), and male infertility.

Diagnosis is suggested by the symptoms and confirmed by imaging (X-ray or CT scan of the paranasal sinuses). Treatment is usually with antibiotics; surgical drainage is occasionally required.

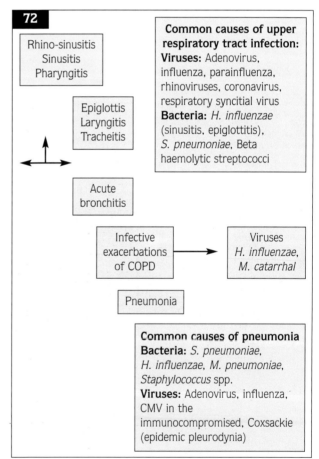

72 Schematic diagram to show infections of the respiratory tract. CMV, cytomegalovirus; COPD, chronic obstructive pulmonary disease

EPIGLOTTITIS

Epiglottitis is a potentially life-threatening condition caused by infection with *H. influenzae* type b. It is commoner in children under 5 years and may present with respiratory distress and painful dysphagia supervening on a history of fever and sore throat. Intrusive examination of the pharynx can cause fatal upper airway obstruction and, should epiglottitis be suspected, upper airway instrumentation should be performed only where facilities for tracheal intubation and tracheostomy are at hand. Treatment in uncomplicated cases is with antibiotics (co-amoxiclav or chloramphenicol). The Hib vaccine, used mainly for the prevention of meningitis, may offer some protection against epiglottitis.

LARYNGOTRACHEOBRONCHITIS

Laryngotracheobronchitis ('croup'), usually due to viruses, is another cause of potentially life-threatening upper respiratory tract infection, usually occurring in children. Steam inhalation and nebulized steroids are of value in the treatment of the stridor that characterizes the severe form of the condition.

PNEUMONIA

Pneumonia is an inflammatory consolidation of the lung parenchyma, usually due to infection but occasionally due to chemical or other insults (**73**). The infecting agents are usually bacteria or viruses, although occasionally, particularly in an immunocompromised host, protozoal and fungal organisms may cause pneumonia. Some of the common causes of pneumonia are shown in *Table 46*.

EPIDEMIOLOGY

The annual incidence of community-acquired pneumonia (CAP) in the United Kingdom is 5–11 per 1,000 of the adult population; the incidence is much higher in the very young and the elderly. Between 22% and 42% of adults with CAP are admitted to hospital and 5–10% of these will require management in the intensive care setting. The overall

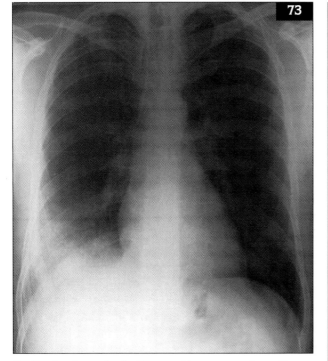

73 Chest radiograph of a 34-year-old man presenting with community-acquired pneumonia showing right lower lobe consolidation

Table 46 Common causes of pneumonia

Bacteria
- ❏ *Streptococcus pneumoniae* (pneumococcus)
- ❏ *Haemophilus influenzae*
- ❏ *Legionella* sp.
- ❏ *Mycoplasma pneumoniae; Chlamydia pneumoniae*
- ❏ Gram-negative bacilli (*Proteus* sp., *E. coli*)
- ❏ *Staphylococcus aureus*
- ❏ *Moraxella catarrhalis*
- ❏ *Chlamydia psittici*
- ❏ *Coxiella burnetti*
- ❏ *Klebsiella pneumoniae*

Viruses
- ❏ Influenza A & B
- ❏ Parainfluenza
- ❏ Cytomegalovirus
- ❏ Adenovirus

Fungi
- ❏ *Aspergillus*
- ❏ *Candida* sp.
- ❏ *Nocardia* sp.
- ❏ *Cryptococcus* sp.
- ❏ *Histoplasma* sp.
- ❏ *Pneumocystis*

mortality for CAP treated in the community is very low (< 1%), rising to 5–12% in those hospitalized with the condition and around 50% in those with severe disease admitted to the intensive care unit. Globally, pneumonia is a common preventable cause of death, particularly among children under the age of 5 years.

PATHOGENESIS AND PATHOLOGY

The lung parenchyma is infiltrated with an inflammatory exudate resulting in the lung tissue losing its elasticity ('consolidation'). In bacterial pneumonia the infiltrate is predominantly neutrophilic, while in viral and parasitic infections it is lymphocytic or mononuclear, or of mixed cellularity.

Table 47 Clinical features of pneumonia

Symptoms
- ❏ Respiratory
  - Cough
  - Sputum (green or rusty)
  - Pleuritic chest pain
  - Breathlessness
  - Occasionally minor haemoptysis
- ❏ Systemic
  - Fever
  - Rigors
  - Headache
  - Muscle pains
  - Anorexia
  - Diarrhoea
  - Collapse

Signs
- ❏ Fever
- ❏ Tachycardia
- ❏ Hypertension
- ❏ Tachypnoea
- ❏ Signs of consolidation (diminished expansion, impaired percussion note, bronchial breathing, pleural rub, crackles, increased vocal fremitus, whispering pectoriloquy)

CLASSIFICATION

Pneumonia can be classified on the basis of:
- ❏ The aetiological agent, e.g. pneumococcal pneumonia, *Mycoplasma* pneumonia, lipoid pneumonia.
- ❏ The clinical presentation symptoms as '*typical*' pneumonia or '*atypical*' (see below), although this classification is of limited value.
- ❏ The setting in which it has occurred – *community-acquired* (CAP) or *hospital-acquired* (*nosocomial*).
- ❏ The immune status of the host – occurring in an *immunocompromised* host (e.g. post bone marrow transplant or HIV) or an *immunocompetent* one. Infections that occur in an immunocompromised host owing to organisms that are normally nonpathogenic are called '*opportunistic infections*'.
- ❏ The anatomical extent of the abnormalities – *lobar*, if the distribution is along a particular lobe or lobes (multi-lobar) or *bronchopneumonia*, if the distribution is along bronchopulmonary segments in one or many lobes. Bronchopneumonia is often the terminal event in the elderly.

CLINICAL FEATURES

The classical symptoms and signs of pneumonia are given in *Table 47*. While some or many of these features may be evident in most patients, in the elderly, diabetics, and the immunocompromised, the problem may not present with typical symptoms or signs and must be actively considered in the context of unexplained general ill-being.

The term 'atypical pneumonia' was used widely in the past to refer to a pneumonic illness – presumed to be due to organisms such as *Mycoplasma pneumoniae* and *Chlamydia* sp. – which often presented as a systemic illness or with symptoms not particularly referable to the respiratory tract (diarrhoea, headache, and so on). It is now accepted that presenting symptoms and signs are not a reliable guide to the agent causing pneumonia.

The salient features of pneumonia caused by various organisms are given in *Table 48*. While these features may help raise suspicion of a particular agent being the cause of the illness, no historical or radiological features can be deemed to be diagnostic and, indeed, history, such as that of occupation or foreign travel, may be misleading.

PNEUMONIA IN THE IMMUNOCOMPROMISED HOST

The spectrum of microbes causing pneumonia is wider in patients with impaired immunity. In addition to the organisms listed above, immunocompromised patients are at risk of infections caused by organisms that are not usually pathogenic and often reside in the respiratory tract as commensals (opportunistic infections). In clinical practice, the following are common groups of patients considered as immunocompromised:

❏ Patients with HIV/acquired immunodeficiency syndrome.

❏ Patients on immunosuppressive drugs (e.g. for vasculitic conditions, RA).

❏ Patients on cytotoxic/chemotherapeutic agents for cancer.

❏ Post bone marrow transplant patients.

❏ Patients with immune paresis due to lymphoma or myeloma.

Patients who have had a splenectomy (surgically or as a result of having a medical condition such as sickle cell disease) are at increased risk of infections by bacteria (Gram-positive cocci).

Table 48 The salient features of pneumonia

Type of pneumonia	Features	Management
Pneumococcal pneumonia (*Streptococcus pneumoniae*) Gram-positive coccus	Commonest cause of CAP (50–60%); classical presentation Tendency to septicaemia High WCC, CRP Tests for pneumococcal antigen in sputum, blood or pleural fluid may help in difficult cases	Amoxicillin; macrolides or levofloxacin (not ciprofloxacin) in patients sensitive to penicillin or resistant areas Pneumococcal vaccination in asplenic patients and others at risk
Mycoplasma pneumonia (*M. pneumoniae*) Pleomorphic organism lacking a cell wall Seasonal (autumn) and 3–4-year cyclical patterns	Less common in the elderly. 'Atypical' presentation with nonpulmonary symptoms and signs (myringitis, arthritis, haemolytic anaemia, erythema multiforme, hepatitis, myocarditis) Serological tests for cold agglutinins and *Mycoplasma titres*	Macrolides or tetracyclines or levofloxacin
Legionella pneumonia (*L. pneumophila*) Gram-negative bacillus Epidemics related to water-containing systems (e.g. cooling towers, shower systems); cluster of cases linked to Mediterranean resorts	Younger patients, smokers, absence of co-morbidity; diarrhoea, neurological symptoms, deranged liver function, hyponatraemia Urine for *Legionella* antigen; serological tests for rising titres	Macrolides or rifampicin or levofloxacin

(continued overleaf)

Table 48 The salient features of pneumonia (continued)

Type of pneumonia	Features	Management
Haemophilus pneumonia (*H. influenzae*) Gram-negative bacillus	In those with pre-existing lung disease; common cause of acute exacerbations of COPD	Amoxicillin Co-amoxiclav in beta lactamase producing cases (10% in the UK), or cefotaxime or cefuroxime or levofloxacin (Hib vaccine provides protection mostly against strains causing meningitis and epiglottitis)
Chlamydia pneumonia (*Chlamydia pneumoniae*) Causes outbreaks in young adults; *Chlamydia psittici* primarily affects birds	Features of 'atypical' pneumonia; hepatitis, renal failure, intravascular coagulation are rare complications	Macrolides or tetracyclines
Staphylococcal pneumonia (*S. aureus*) Gram-positive coccus Commoner during influenza epidemics; occasionally due to MRSA	Rare cause of CAP in the UK Cavitating pneumonia; may be associated with serious systemic illness	Flucloxacillin. Vancomycin for MRSA
Gram-negative bacilli (*Pseudomonas aeruginosa*; *Escherichia coli*; *Klebsiella pneumoniae*) More commonly cause nosocomial pneumonia; *Klebsiella* is commoner in the elderly and in alcoholics	Typical pneumonic symptoms and signs but may be less evident in the elderly Mortality higher on account of co-morbidity and age	Cefuroxime, cefotaxime or ceftriaxone Imipenem Ceftazidime for *Pseudomonas*
Q fever (*Coxiella burnetti*) Rickettsial organism transmitted by ticks on domestic cattle, sheep (NB occupational history)	Usually benign course; commoner in lambing and calving season Nonspecific clinical features	Tetracycline or macrolides
Rarer pneumonias		
Pneumonic plague (*Yersinia pestis*) Transmitted by flea bites or person-to-person	Pneumonic plague presents with cough, dyspnoea, haemoptysis; radiographic changes of pneumonia	Pneumonic plague Tetracyclines; streptomycin
Anthrax (*Bacillus anthracis*)	Nonproductive cough, chest pain, dyspnoea, stridor; X-ray may show pleural effusions and enlargement of the mediastinum	Anthrax Penicillins; tetracycline macrolides;chloramphenico.l
Chickenpox pneumonia (varicella zoster)	Commoner in smoking adults and pregnant women; respiratory symptoms may develop 5–7 days after the rash	Chickenpox (varicella) Acyclovir

CAP, community-acquired pneumonia; COPD, chronic obstructive pulmonary disease; CRP, C-reactive protein; MRSA, methicillin-resistant *Staphylococcus aureus*; WCC, white cell count

Clinical features

In the immmunocompromised host pneumonia may not present with symptoms referable to the respiratory system, although a dry cough and breathlessness on exertion are common presenting symptoms. Likewise, the brisk immune response seen in the immuno-competent adult, leading to leucocytosis and an elevated CRP, may not be evident. Any unexplained ill-being or fever in an immunocompromised host should prompt a careful examination of the respiratory system and a request for a chest radiograph. *Table 49* describes the commoner causes of pneumonia in the immunocompromised host and the clinical features of the illness.

INVESTIGATIONS AND DIAGNOSIS

In general, patients with CAP mild enough to be managed in the community do not require a radiological confirmation of the illness, nor the other investigations detailed below. Failure to respond to therapy should prompt consideration of micro-biological investigations, including sputum examination and culture (including for TB). Serological testing for *Legionella* or *Mycoplasma* may be considered during suspected outbreaks.

Table 49 Pneumonia in the immunocompromised host

Infection	Clinical features	Treatment
Pneumocystis jiroveci pneumonia (formerly *P. carinii*) (PCP) Until recently believed to be protozoan; now thought to be a fungus Demonstrated by Giemsa or silver staining and immunofluorescence techniques	Patients with a CD4 count of < 200/mm^3 at risk Dry cough, breathlessness In the early stages chest radiograph may be normal; later, progression from perihilar ('bat's wings') shadowing to extensive bilateral interstitial shadowing Diagnosis by demonstrating organism in sputum (if necessary induced with nebulized saline), BAL fluid or biopsy (**74**)	High dose trimethoprim – co-trimoxazole (Septrin) Oral Septrin or nebulized pentamidine used as prophylaxis
Aspergillus pneumonia (*A. fumigatus*) Fungal organism; acquired from the environment Demonstrated by Groccott staining	Invasive pulmonary aspergillosis is common, particularly in bone marrow transplant patients and lymphoma patients Demonstration in respiratory secretions cannot distinguish between colonization and invasive infection; demonstration of organism in tissue is ideal	Ambisome: liposomes of amphotericin phospholipids (less nephrotoxic than amphotericin B)
Cytomegalovirus Serological conversion (cytomegalovirus antibody) and demonstration of 'owl-eye' intranuclear inclusion bodies in lung biopsy specimens	Commoner in conditions associated with T-cell suppression (especially post transplant); seronegative patients at risk if they receive transplants from seropositive donors Nonspecific symptoms, signs, and radiological features	Ganciclovir, foscarnet, ribavarin Ganciclovir can be used as a prophylactic agent

All patients hospitalized with CAP should have the following investigations as a minimum: chest radiograph, full blood count, urea, electrolytes, liver function tests, CRP, and pulse oximetry. A summary of the investigations available in the management of CAP is shown in *Table 50*.

Serum chemistry

Blood urea measurements help with diagnosis (see below); CRP is elevated in bacterial infections and serial measurements are helpful in charting the response to treatment. Hyponatraemia is a well recognized feature of *Legionella* pneumonia, although any severe pneumonia can cause the syndrome of inappropriate ADH secretion (SIADH).

Full blood count

A full blood count usually reveals a neutrophilic leucocytosis; leucopenia (white cell count $< 4 \times 10^9/l$) is associated with a poorer outcome. Mycoplasma pneumonia can be associated with a haemolytic anaemia. The presence of marked eosinophilia must raise the suspicion of an alternative diagnosis, e.g. cryptogenic eosinophilic pneumonia or Churg–Strauss syndrome.

Chest radiograph

A chest radiograph may show typical pneumonic consolidation in one or more lobes (**74**). It is important to bear in mind that radiological changes lag behind clinical status, with shadowing in the lung fields worsening in the face of clinical improvement. Radiological abnormalities may take 4–6 weeks (even longer in the elderly) to resolve. In addition to confirming the diagnosis, a chest radiograph also helps in the identification of co-existing cardiorespiratory disease (e.g. heart failure, bronchiectasis) and the onset of complications (e.g. parapneumonic effusion, empyema, lung abscess, and so on).

More advanced imaging, in particular CT scanning of the thorax, is considered only in cases where an alternative diagnosis – including underlying lung cancer – merits serious consideration. It is not necessary to repeat a chest radiograph prior to discharge or on any other occasion to confirm improvement, except in patients in whom there has been incomplete recovery clinically (persistent symptoms and physical signs) and/or where there is concern regarding the possibitiy of underlying lung cancer (smokers > 50 years of age).

Table 50 Summary of investigations available in the management of community-acquired pneumonia

- ❏ Chest radiograph
- ❏ Full blood count
- ❏ Blood urea and electrolytes
- ❏ C-reactive protein
- ❏ Pulse oximetry: arterial blood gas analysis
- ❏ Blood culture
- ❏ Sputum examination (Gram staining; examination for acid-fast bacilli) and culture
- ❏ Paired serological tests (*Mycoplasma, Legionella*)
- ❏ Urinary antigen for *Legionella*
- ❏ Bronchoalveolar lavage; culture of lower respiratory tract secretions obtained by a protected brush biopsy on bronchoscopy

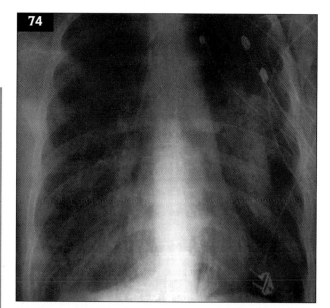

74 Chest radiograph of a 43-year-old homosexual male presenting with weight loss and dyspnoea. Bronchoalveolar lavage helped in the diagnosis of pneumocystis pneumonia (PCP). Note the presence of a pneumothorax and intercostal drains. Pneumothorax is a well recognized complication of PCP. Tests for HIV were positive in this patient

Oxygen saturations and arterial blood gas analysis

Pulse oximetry is a useful screening test to identify the risk of respiratory failure and the need to perform an arterial puncture for blood gas analysis. An SaO_2 of < 92%, breathing room air, indicates the need for full blood gas analysis and supplementary oxygen therapy. Blood gas analysis, in patients with no co-existing COPD or other respiratory illnesses, usually reveals a type I respiratory failure, with hypoxaemia and normal or low arterial carbon dioxide levels. Arterial gas analysis also aids in decisions regarding ventilatory support (see Chapter 13, page 130).

Microbiological investigations and identification of the causative organism

While attempts are routinely made to identify the organism causing pneumonia, it is arguable whether the results of these investigations make a difference to the overall outcomes in uncomplicated disease. A full range of microbiological investigations is therefore not recommended in all patients with pneumonia. The pursuit of a bacteriological diagnosis is dictated by the severity and context of the illness and the response to treatment, and is particularly relevant in initial treatment failures and in immunocompromised patients.

It is recommended that all patients hospitalized with CAP undergo blood culture and that sputum culture is also performed in patients who are productive of sputum. Gram-staining of the sputum may be valuable in patients with severe CAP, in whom it may guide early empirical treatment (see below).

Serological tests

Serological tests are useful in the diagnosis of 'atypical' pneumonia (*Legionella* and *Mycoplasma*). A fourfold rise in antibody titres in the serum of a convalescent patient, demonstrated by paired serological tests, provides retrospective evidence of infection by these organisms. It is recommended that serological tests are carried out in all patients with severe CAP, in patients failing to respond to aminopenicillin, and for epidemiological reasons during specific outbreaks. Demonstration of seroconversion to cytomegalovirus (CMV) may be useful corroborative evidence of CMV pneumonitis in an immunocompromised host. Tests are available for the detection of *Legionella* antigens in urine and pneumococcal antigens in various body fluids (including pleural fluid) and secretions.

Bronchoalveolar lavage (BAL) and sampling of lower respiratory secretions by a protected brush via a bronchoscope (to prevent contamination by upper airway and oral commensals) are techniques employed, usually in an immunocompromised host, to secure specimens for microbiological examination. Gram staining, staining for acid-fast bacilli, and silver staining for *Pneumocystis* are routinely performed on such specimens, as is culture in a wide range of media (including for TB and *Legionella*). When used judiciously and before empirical multi-agent or broad-spectrum antibiotic therapy, BAL is a valuable tool in the management of pneumonia occurring in an immunocompromised host (74). Even in patients investigated extensively, a microbiological diagnosis may be secured in only < 40% of cases.

DIFFERENTIAL DIAGNOSIS OF PNEUMONIA

Table 51 shows the differential diagnosis of pneumonia.

MANAGEMENT

CAP can usually be treated in an outpatient setting. The presence of two or more of the core adverse prognostic features or one of these features in a patient older than 50 years or with pre-existing lung disease (see below) should prompt consideration of hospitalization, as should poor social circumstances, particularly in the elderly.

Table 51 The differential diagnoses of pneumonia

❏ Bronchitis

❏ Infective exacerbations of chronic obstructive pulmonary disease

❏ Pulmonary oedema

❏ Pulmonary infarction (pulmonary thromboembolic disease)

❏ Lung cancer

❏ Extrinsic allergic alveolitis

❏ Asthma

❏ Other parenchymal lung diseases:

Eosinophilic pneumonia

Cryptogenic organizing pneumonitis

Drug-induced lung disease

Antibiotic therapy in CAP

Empirical antibiotic therapy should not await the results of investigations but be commenced immediately if there is a suspicion of CAP. Most patients with CAP can be treated in the community and with oral antibiotics. In patients referred to hospital, where there is likely to be a delay (> 2 hrs) in admission or in those with life-threatening illness, the general practitioner may consider administering an antibiotic before transfer to hospital. While there may be variations in the antibiotics chosen as empirical first-line therapy in CAP, there are some general principles that underlie this treatment (*Table 52*).

Table 52 General principles of management of community-acquired pneumonia (CAP)

❏ Any empirical therapy for CAP should be effective against *Streptococcus pneumoniae*, which is the most common cause of CAP (even in those in whom no organism is isolated)

❏ In the UK amoxicillin at a dose of 500 mg thrice daily is the preferred agent; a macrolide (erythromycin or clarithromycin) can be used in patients with penicillin allergy

❏ In hospitalized patients a combination of an aminopenicillin and a macrolide is preferred

❏ Amoxicillin monotherapy may suffice in patients who have previously been untreated in the community and in the elderly, in whom 'atypical' pathogens (resistant to penicillins and responsive to macrolides) are uncommon

❏ Fluoroquinolones active against *S. pneumoniae* (e.g. levofloxacin) can be used as monotherapy; ciprofloxacin is ineffective against *S. pneumoniae* and should not be used as a first-line agent for empirical treatment of CAP

❏ Most patients can be effectively treated with oral antibiotics; IV antibiotics are used only in hospitalized patients with severe pneumonia, loss of consciousness, impaired swallowing or malabsorption

❏ In immunocompromised patients empirical therapy may include high-dose trimethoprim/sulphonamide (e.g. Septrin) (for pneumocystis pneumonia) and ganciclovir (cytomegalovirus pneumonia) as well as antifungal agents (liposomal amphotericin for *Aspergillus* infection)

❏ Empirical antibiotic therapy should be reviewed if there are no signs of improvement or if a pathogen has been identified and is recognized as being resistant to the antibiotic therapy being given

---

Supportive treatment

All patients with pneumonia should be advised not to smoke. Adequate hydration must be ensured, if necessary intravenously in the severely ill and unconscious. Adequate analgesia must be provided. Hypoxia and respiratory failure should be managed along recommended lines by appropriate use of oxygen therapy and ventilatory support (Chapter 13, page 131).

COMPLICATIONS OF PNEUMONIA

Table 53 shows the complications of pneumonia.

NATURAL HISTORY AND PROGNOSIS IN PNEUMONIA

The vast majority of patients with CAP recover uneventfully, but the outcome in nosocomial pneumonias is less satisfactory. Recovery may be slow to occur in the elderly, particularly those with multi-lobe involvement (*Table 54*). Radiological improvement often lags behind symptomatic improvement.

Failure to improve with treatment in pneumonia can be due to:
❏ Wrong diagnosis (*Table 51*, page 109):
   – Foreign bodies, particularly in children.
   – Lung cancer in smoking adults.
   – TB in relevant 'at-risk' groups.
❏ Wrong treatment:
   – Inappropriate empirical therapy (e.g. ciprofloxacin as first-line treatment for CAP).
   – Oral therapy in the presence of vomiting or diarrhoea.
   – Failure to use adequate doses of antibiotics.
❏ Antibiotic resistance.
❏ Onset of complications (*Table 53*).

Table 53 Complications of pneumonia

❏ Parapneumonic effusion

❏ Empyema (see Chapter 9, page 95)

❏ Lung abscess (see Chapter 11, page 121)

❏ Respiratory failure (see Chapter 13, page 128)

❏ Acute respiratory distress syndrome

❏ Septic shock; multiple organ system failure

❏ Cryptogenic organizing pneumonia

❏ Bronchiectasis (late complication)

❏ Pneumococcal pneumonia may be associated with acute endicarditis and meningitis

SPECIFIC PNEUMONIA PROBLEMS
Aspiration pneumonia

Aspiration pneumonia may occur in the context of states of diminished consciousness (e.g. seizures, anaesthesia, alcoholic stupor) when oropharyngeal, oesophageal or gastric contents are aspirated into the respiratory tract. A chemical pneumonitis and/or bacterial infection (anaerobic bacteria: *Bacteroides* sp., *Fusobacterium*) results. Lipoid pneumonia (caused by aspiration of exogenous lipid material, usually laxatives or nasal decongestant medication) is a form of aspiration pneumonia, and near-drowning can present as an aspiration pneumonia. Antibiotics given for aspiration pneumonia must be effective against anaerobes (penicillin, metronidazole). Care is needed to prevent aspiration in circumstances predisposing to it (lateral decubitus during seizure activity, nasogastric intubation in states of unconsciousness, and so on).

Nosocomial pneumonia

Hospital-acquired, or nosocomial pneumonia (NP), accounts for around 15% of all infections acquired in hospital and is the second most common cause of nosocomial infections (after infections of the urinary tract). At-risk patients include those undergoing major, particularly abdominal, surgery and those with multiple organ failure. The risk of NP is higher in those admitted to the intensive care unit, where as many as 50% of patients receiving ventilation suffer from the condition.

> **Table 54 Predictors of poor outcome in pneumonia**
>
> **Core features** (CURB-65)
>
> **C**onfusion: minimental score of 8 or less
>
> **U**rea: > 7 mmol/l
>
> **R**espiratory rate: > 30 / min
>
> **B**lood pressure: systolic < 90 mmHg; diastolic < 60 mmHg
>
> **65:** Age > 65 years
>
> **Additional adverse features**
>
> ❑ Pre-existing: age 50 years and above; presence of co-existing disease (cardiac, respiratory, renal, and other)
>
> ❑ Hypoxaemia (SaO_2 < 92% or PaO_2 < 8 kPa)
>
> ❑ White cell count of > 20 or < 4 x 10^9/l
>
> ❑ Bilateral or multi-lobe involvement
>
> ❑ A positive blood culture

The mortality from NP is considerably higher than that from CAP, with NP accounting for as many as 10% of all deaths in hospital.

NP differs from CAP in that the causative organisms are mainly Gram-negative bacteria (*Pseudomonas* sp., *Proteus* sp., *Escherichia coli*, and so on) or, if Gram-positive, organisms that are likely to be resistant to penicillins (including MRSA – methicillin-resistant *Staphylococcus aureus*).

Empirical therapy for the condition differs from that for CAP, with ceftazidime being the preferred antibiotic for pseudomonal NP, while other third-generation cephalosporins (cefuroxime or cefotaxime) and/or aminoglycosides or quinolones (e.g. ciprofloxacin) are preferred for other Gram-negative organisms, and intravenous vancomycin for MRSA. Broader spectrum agents like imipenem are also used.

PREVENTION OF PNEUMONIA

The Department of Health recommends pneumococcal vaccination for all those aged 2 years or over in whom pneumococcal infection is likely to be more common or serious (post-splenectomy patients, diabetics, those with co-existing heart failure, COPD or renal failure). The vaccine should not be administered during pregnancy or an acute infection. Re-immunization is not required for 4 years. The influenza and pneumococcal vaccines can be administered at the same time (at different sites).

TUBERCULOSIS

TB is a disease caused by the organism *Mycobacterium tuberculosis*. *Mycobacterium bovis*, endemic in cattle and spread through infected milk, was an occasional cause of human TB in previous years, but TB in humans now is almost exclusively due to *M. tuberculosis*. There are a number of species of saprophytes belonging to the genus *Mycobacterium* (e.g. *M. kansasii*, *M. avium intracellulare*) that do not normally cause disease in man. These environmental mycobacteria (previously called atypical mycobacteria or opportunistic mycobacteria) cause disease only in immunocompromised subjects or those with pre-existing lung disease; the disease caused by these organisms is not labelled tuberculosis.

EPIDEMIOLOGY

Worldwide, nearly 2 billion people – one third of the world's population – are infected with *Mycobacterium tuberculosis* and 8 million new cases of the disease occur each year. Over 95% of the new cases occur in the developing world, as do over 95% of the 3 million deaths per year that are caused by the disease. In 1993 the WHO declared TB a global emergency.

In the UK the incidence of TB showed a tendency to a gradual decline over the earlier part of the 20th century (75), but there has been a small but perceptible reversal of this trend over the last 15 years. In 1998, in England and Wales, there were 6,572 new cases of TB (73% pulmonary) and 392 deaths due to the condition.

The disease affects the ethnic minority population disproportionately, with incidence rates 50 times higher in persons of Black African origin and 40 times higher in those of Bangladeshi, Indian, and Pakistani origin, compared with the white population (76). In addition to patients from certain ethnic minorities, the homeless, alcohol dependent, and immunocompromised patients are considered to be at a higher than average risk of suffering from TB. Most TB in the UK occurs among people living in the inner cities (76). Disease rates in London, in particular, are high and have doubled in the past 10 years.

PATHOGENESIS AND PATHOLOGY

Mycobacterium tuberculosis is spread by person-to-person droplet infection, usually via the respiratory tract. Only 10% or less of persons infected by the bacillus develop disease. In a small proportion of cases the initial infection may directly progress to disease, usually of the lung. The 'primary complex' of the disease is made up of a lesion in the lungs and accompanying disease in the mediastinal or hilar lymph nodes. Haematogenous spread can result in the disease affecting other sites, with symptoms manifesting years after the initial infection. Most new cases seen in clinical practice in adults are due to reactivation of previously dormant infection, rather than newly acquired infection. The term 'miliary TB' is applied to the extensive disease that occurs in the elderly or malnourished subject, involving multiple organs (lungs, liver, and so on), and often presenting with characteristic chest radiograph appearances (see below).

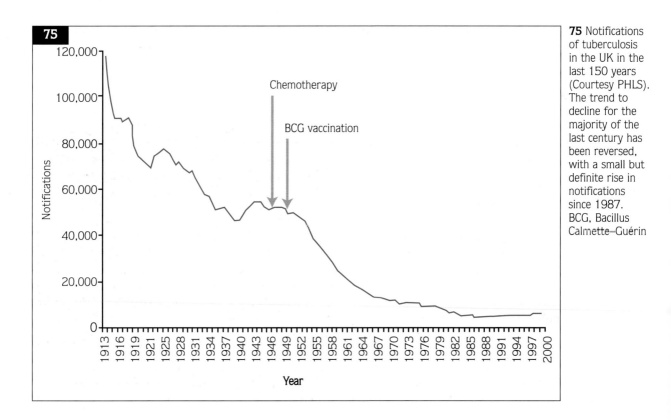

75 Notifications of tuberculosis in the UK in the last 150 years (Courtesy PHLS). The trend to decline for the majority of the last century has been reversed, with a small but definite rise in notifications since 1987. BCG, Bacillus Calmette–Guérin

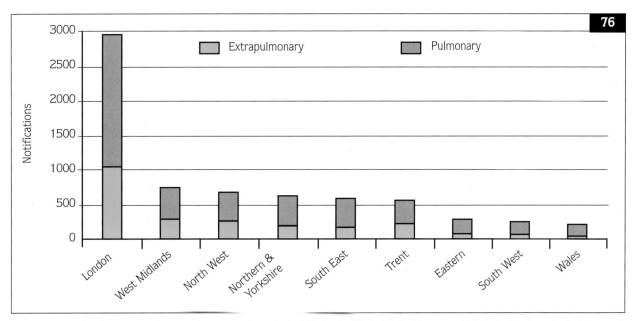

76 Incidence of pulmonary and extrapulmonary tuberculosis (TB) in the UK in 2000 (Courtesy PHLS). In London, the incidence of TB equals that of many developing nations

A caseating granuloma is the characteristic histopathological abnormality evident on examination of tissue affected by TB. The granuloma comprises chronic inflammatory cells including lymphocytes and multinucleate giant cells and the caseation represents an area of focal necrosis.

CLINICAL FEATURES
Fever, night sweats, weight loss, and general malaise are often the striking presenting symptoms, in addition to the symptoms related to the organ system affected by the disease.

Pleuropulmonary TB
This is the commonest manifestation of TB. The usual symptoms are cough, sputum production, and, less commonly, haemoptysis. Breathlessness may be a feature, particularly in patients with a sizeable pleural effusion. Physical examination may reveal a pleural effusion, features of focal fibrosis (usually of the upper lobe) or, occasionally, lobar collapse in some patients with lymph node disease in the mediastinum or hila causing bronchial obstruction. Physical examination of the chest may be normal even in patients with extensive radiological abnormalities.

A chest radiograph may reveal typical features (77) of upper lobe shadowing with or without cavitation. Pleural effusions and hilar or mediastinal lymphadenopathy are often evident. In miliary TB (*milia* = millet seed) both lung fields are filled with small nodular opacities < 5 mm in diameter distributed uniformly over all lobes.

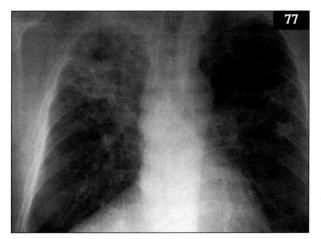

77 Chest radiograph of an immigrant from Burma, presenting with cough, sputum, and weight loss. Note the upper lobe preponderance of the opacities and the tendency to cavitation, indicating active disease

Nonpulmonary manifestations of TB

TB can affect virtually any organ system but some are affected more commonly than others. The commoner nonpulmonary manifestations of TB are listed below:

❏ *TB lymphadenitis* : more common among patients from the Indian sub-continent; accounts for 25% or more of all cases of extrapulmonary TB; commonly affects cervical and mediastinal lymph nodes.

❏ *Genito-urinary TB:* accounts for 15% of nonpulmonary TB. TB granuloma of the kidneys and bladder (resulting in scarring and 'thimble bladder'); may present with sterile pyuria; TB epididymitis and prostatitis.

❏ *Bone TB:* Pott's disease of the spine is due to TB affecting the vertebrae; can result in cord compression causing paraplegia; may present as paraspinal 'cold' abscesses (so called owing to the absence of signs of acute inflammation) which in the thoracolumbar region can track along the psoas muscle to the abdomen and inguinal area; chronic osteomyelitis in any bone.

❏ *Central nervous system (CNS) TB:* meningitis (5% of extrapulmonary TB) may present with headache, confusion, seizures, and personality changes; cerebrospinal fluid (CSF) shows lymphocytic pleocytosis, elevated protein levels with AFB on examination (25%) or culture (> 60%); associated with a mortality of about 20%; early diagnosis and treatment associated with better outcomes; tuberculomas (TB granulomas) in the CNS may cause symptoms of a space-occupying lesion (headache, vomiting, or signs of raised intracranial tension). Steroid therapy may be useful in some cases of CNS disease.

❏ *Abdominal TB:* TB peritonitis and ileocaecal TB (presenting as an 'appendix mass' or as a sinus in the abdominal wall).

❏ *Cutaneous TB:* erythema induratum, lupus vulgaris.

❏ *TB pericarditis.*

INVESTIGATIONS AND DIAGNOSIS

Tuberculin testing

The immune response (type IV – delayed hypersensitivity) to tubercle bacilli is determined by the cutaneous response to an intradermal injection of a TB bacillus-derived protein (purified protein derivative [PPD]). In the *Mantoux* test variable concentrations of PPD are injected intradermally with a syringe on the volar surface of the nondominant arm and the area of induration (not erythema) that develops around the injection site is measured 48–72 hours later. In the *Heaf test* a spring-loaded gun is used to inject a fixed amount of PPD intradermally in a circular pattern, and the reaction is graded as I–IV depending on the response. Interpretation of the response to the tuberculin test should take into account the age of the subject and Bacillus Calmette–Guérin (BCG) vaccination status (BCG vaccination results in a mildly positive tuberculin response). Even a mildly positive response in a child who has not received BCG should raise the suspicion of primary infection. A strong tuberculin response (grade 3–4 Heaf) in an adult, regardless of BCG status, should prompt a thorough assessment for evidence of disease, while the upgrading of a response in an asymptomatic contact of a case of TB should prompt consideration of chemoprophylaxis (see below).

Bacteriological diagnosis

The presence of tubercle bacilli is demonstrated by the Ziehl–Neelsen technique (staining with carbol-fuschin red dye that is not washed out by acid or alcohol – hence the term acid- or alcohol-fast bacillus [AFB]). Culture of the specimen in a special medium (Lowenstein–Jensen) takes 6–8 weeks and helps characterize the organism further, particularly its sensitivity to the various anti-tuberculous drugs. More recent culture techniques (Bactec 460®) enable earlier (1–3 weeks) identification of the organism.

Polymerase chain reaction (PCR) based techniques to detect the tubercle bacillus are of value in some circumstances (e.g. in the diagnosis of TB meningitis) where the bacterial load is low and staining for AAFB may be negative. DNA probes for detecting particular strains of the bacilli are used to detect early the presence of drug-resistant TB, in particular resistance to rifampicin.

Sputum, early morning urine, CSF, and pleural fluid are among the common specimens that are examined for AAFB. In general at least three separate samples of the specimen, provided on three consecutive days, are examined. In patients with suspected pulmonary TB in whom there is no sputum production, a bronchoscopy and a BAL of the radiologically affected lobe of the lung may reveal AAFB.

Histological examination
Histological examination of tissue may reveal a caseating granuloma with or without acid-fast bacilli.

MANAGEMENT OF TB
Notification
TB is a notifiable disease and the diagnosis, even in the absence of bacteriological confirmation, should be notified to the public health department (Centres of Communicable Diseases Control [CCDC]). The local respiratory physician should be involved in the management of the condition, even in patients with extrapulmonary disease.

Contact tracing and infectivity
Cases whose sputum is positive for AAFB on staining ('sputum smear positive') are considered most infectious. Pulmonary TB patients whose sputum is smear negative but culture positive are considered less at risk of transmitting the disease, while those with nonpulmonary TB are generally considered noninfectious. Patients who are sputum smear positive are considered noninfectious after 2 weeks of anti-TB treatment. Although hospitalization and isolation of smear positive patients are not mandatory (except in those suspected of multidrug resistant disease), they are generally recommended.

Contact tracing is performed: to identify cases of TB associated with the index case; to identify persons who have been infected but do not exhibit evidence of disease; and to detect a source of infection (particularly in children). In general, close contacts (partner, members of the same household) of cases with pulmonary disease are screened with a tuberculin test and, if appropriate, a chest radiograph. In patients who show strong evidence of infection but no disease, chemoprophylaxis (see below) may be of value.

DRUG THERAPY
Antituberculous chemotherapy is extremely effective and when recommended treatment regimes are adhered to, the chances of relapse are < 3%. The following general principles apply:

❏ Isoniazid (INH) and rifampicin are the key anti-tuberculous agents. The standard regime comprises four drugs – INH, rifampicin, pyrazinamide, and ethambutol – given for 2 months followed by two drugs (INH and rifampicin) for 4 months. In patients at low risk of drug resistance (Caucasian origin with no previous treatment for TB), three drugs (INH, rifampicin, and pyrazinamide) may be used for the first 2 months.

❏ Except for TB of the central nervous system (TB meningitis or tuberculoma), where the treatment is continued for 12 months, a 6-month regime is sufficient.

❏ Resistance to any one of the main agents (INH or rifampicin) results in prolongation of the treatment with the other drugs, usually making for a total of 9 months or more of treatment.

❏ The drugs are all given in a once daily dose to be taken on an empty stomach 30 minutes before breakfast; for convenience proprietary preparations, containing a combination of INH, rifampicin, and pyrazinamide, and INH and rifampicin are available.

❏ The conventional first-line treatment is safe in pregnant and breast-feeding women.

❏ Multi-drug resistant TB (resistant to INH and rifampicin) is four times more common in HIV patients.

Listed in *Table 55* are the commonly used anti-tuberculous drugs and their side-effects.

Directly observed therapy (DOT)

This is the term applied to anti-TB treatment where the ingestion of every drug dose is witnessed by a health care worker or a designated carer. Worldwide, the WHO recommends this as the standard procedure on the grounds that failure to comply voluntarily with the recommended therapy is one of the main reasons for poor outcomes from TB. However in situations where concordance with therapy is likely to be greater than 90%, routine use of DOT regimes may be inappropriate. In the UK, DOT is considered only in patient who are homeless, mentally ill, those with alcohol dependence, patients with multidrug resistant TB, those with a previous history of noncompliance, and in new immigrants and refugees. Patients who have relapsed may also be candidates for DOT.

PREVENTION OF TB
BCG vaccination

BCG is a vaccine containing a live attenuated strain of *M. bovis*. In the UK the national policy is that BCG should be offered to those children and other certain groups at higher risk of exposure to TB (infants and children of immigrants, children born in the UK to parents from ethnic minorities, and healthcare professionals). Neonates and infants up to the age of 3 months can be given BCG without tuberculin testing but, in older children, Heaf testing, to demonstrate a negative immune response, must be performed before immunization.

It is generally accepted that BCG provides 75% protection against the disease for a period of about 15 years. The protective effect is stronger for TB meningitis than pulmonary disease. There is very little evidence to suggest that BCG offers protection when given to people over the age of 16.

Table 55 Anti-tuberculous drugs

Drug	Features
INH (Isoniazid) Usual dose in adults: 300 mg once daily	Bactericidal; first-line treatment; given for entire 6 months; resistance commoner in patients with HIV and those from Indian sub-continent Side-effects: peripheral neuropathy (preventable with pyridoxine); hepatitis; hypersensitivity (rash)
Rifampicin Usual dose in adults: 600 mg once daily	Bactericidal; first-line treatment; resistance rare except in HIV patients; given for entire 6 months Interacts with oral contraceptives and other medications metabolized by the liver Side-effects: colours urine and body fluids orange; hepatitis; thrombocytopenia; 'flu syndrome'; hypersensitivity
Pyrazinamide Usual dose in adults: 15 mg/ kg body weight once daily	Bactericidal (particularly active against intracellular organisms); given for the first 2 months of the 6-month course (longer if INH or rifampicin resistant) Side-effects: hepatotoxicity; hyperuricaemia; hypersensitivity
Ethambutol Usual dose in adults: 15 mg/ kg body weight once daily	Bacteriostatic; given for the first 2 months of the 6-month course (longer if INH or rifampicin resistant) Eye testing (visual acuity) mandatory before commencing treatment Side-effects: optic neuritis (particularly in patients with renal disease)
Streptomycin Usual dose in adults: 15 mg/kg body weight (IM)	Bactericidal; second-line drug; contraindicated in pregnancy Side-effects: auditory and vestibular toxicity; renal impairment
Other second-line agents: ethionamide, prothionamide, para amino salicylic acid (PAS), clarithromycin, ciprofloxacin	These are used only in the presence of resistance to one or more of the first-line agents or severe intolerance (hepatic side-effects or hypersensitivity) to the first-line agents. Which agent is used is dictated by the sensitivity profile of the organism

Chemoprophylaxis

INH for 6 months or INH and rifampicin for 3 months are given to some contacts with a strong tuberculin reaction with no radiological or clinical evidence of disease. The risks of developing the disease must be weighed against the small but definite risk of drug-induced hepatitis from the chemprophylactic drugs.

Screening of immigrants

The incidence of TB in the immigrant population is highest in the first few years after entry into the UK and is usually due to reactivation rather than re-infection. Current recommendations are that all immigrants from countries other than those of the European Union, Canada, United States, Australia, and New Zealand are screened, usually in the immigrant's intended district of residence. Screening consists of a health status interview, including current symptoms, previous tuberculosis, and previous BCG vaccination. Tuberculin testing and further investigations are performed as appropriate.

ENVIRONMENTAL MYCOBACTERIAL INFECTIONS

Environmental mycobacteria are saprophytic organisms that do not cause disease except in patients with pre-existing lung conditions (e.g. COPD, bronchiectasis) or a compromised immune status (e.g. HIV). The organisms (M. kansasii, M. avium-intracellulare [MAI], M. xenopi, and so on) are acid and alcohol fast (AFB) and cause a clinical picture similar to that of TB but with less systemic upset; the disease is not notifiable. Lung disease and lymph node disease are commonest; disseminated MAI infections occur in HIV patients. Treatment regimes usually include rifampicin and ethambutol and need to be continued for 9–24 months (and in some cases indefinitely).

HUMAN IMMUNODEFICIENCY VIRUS

HIV AND TB

- Worldwide, a third of the 36 million people living with HIV are co-infected with TB; in sub-Saharan Africa 70% of TB patients are HIV positive.
- It is estimated that in London about 10% of patients with TB may be co-infected with HIV.
- Classic presentation of TB is less common in HIV patients (lower lobe disease, no pyrexia).
- Low CD4 counts predispose to disseminated TB.
- HIV positivity is associated with a fourfold risk of multi-drug resistant TB (MDR-TB).
- Anti-retroviral treatment can, paradoxically, make the symptoms and signs of TB worse.

HIV AND THE LUNG

The involvement of the lung in HIV can be related to either infectious or noninfectious conditions.

Pulmonary infections in HIV

In addition to the various organisms causing CAP in the immunocompetent individual (see above), patients with HIV are also at risk of opportunistic infection (Table 49, page 107). Important among the pulmonary infections in HIV are infections due to:

- Bacteria: S. pneumoniae, H. influenzae, S. aureus, Nocardia sp., Pseudomonas.
- Fungi : Pneumocystis carinii, Cryptococcus, Aspergillus, Candida, Histoplasma.
- Viruses: cytomegalovirus, herpes simplex, varicella zoster.
- Mycobacteria (M. tuberculosis and environmental, particularly Mycobacterium avium-intracellulare).
- Parasites: Toxoplasma, Cryptosporidium, Microsporidium, Strongyloides.

Although some radiological features are very suggestive of infection by certain organisms (e.g. 'bat's wing' appearance of Pneumocystis, 'coin lesion' of Nocardia), a reliable bacteriological diagnosis is often not achieved without invasive investigations (BAL and transbronchial lung biopsy). Examination of induced sputum may sometimes obviate the need for invasive investigations.

Oxygen desaturation on exercise, as demonstrated by pulse oximetry, is a useful and sensitive, if nonspecific, noninvasive test in the early diagnosis of lung disease in HIV patients.

Noninfectious pulmonary disease in HIV

The common noninfectious complications of HIV disease of the lungs are:

- Nonmalignant:
  - Lymphocytic interstitial pneumonitis.
  - Nonspecific interstitial pneumonitis.
  - Bronchiolitis obiliterans organizing pneumonia (BOOP).
  - Idiopathic pulmonary hypertension.
- Malignant:
  - Kaposi's sarcoma.
  - Non-Hodgkin's lymphoma.
  - Hodgkin's lymphoma.
  - Lung cancer.

The presentation is often insidious and the diagnosis usually requires a lung biopsy, either transbronchial or an open lung biopsy. The outlook for malignant conditions in the context of HIV is much poorer in comparison with the same condition occurring in a non-HIV patient (e.g. median survival for HIV patients with non-Hodgkin's lymphoma is only 6.5 months compared with over 2 years in non-HIV patients).

SUMMARY

❏ Respiratory tract infections are an extremely common cause of ill health and account for around 10% of all consultations in general practice.

❏ Most upper respiratory tract infections are self-limiting but epiglottitis and croup can cause life-threatening upper airway obstruction.

❏ Infective exacerbations of COPD and pneumonia are the common lower respiratory tract infections.

❏ CAP affects 5–10 adults per 1,000 population each year in the UK, the disease being commoner in the very young and the elderly. About a third of patients with the disease are hospitalized. Mortality from the condition is very low at < 1%, increasing to around 8% in hospitalized patients and to 50% in those admitted to the intensive care unit.

❏ Hospital-acquired (nosocomial) pneumonia has a poorer outlook, particularly in the elderly, and is more likely to be caused by Gram-negative agents.

❏ Confusion, blood urea levels, respiratory rate, and blood pressure (CURB) measurements help in identifying those at risk of dying from pneumonia.

❏ In most cases empirical antibiotic therapy is given while investigations for identification of a specific pathogen are pursued. Any empirical therapy for CAP should be effective against *Pneumococcus*, which is the commonest cause of CAP.

❏ Pneumonia in an immunocompromised host (HIV, cancer chemotherapy, post transplant, and so on) can be due to fungal or viral organisms that do not usually cause serious disease in man (e.g. *Pneumocystis*, *Aspergillus* and cytomegalovirus).

❏ TB is a common and serious problem worldwide, causing 3 million deaths each year.

❏ In the UK, after a century of decreasing incidence, TB is on the rise, particularly in London.

❏ Patients from ethnic minorities, the immunocompromised, the homeless, and the alcohol dependent are at higher risk of the disease, which affects mainly the lungs but can also affect other organs (extrapulmonary TB).

❏ Treatment of TB is for at least 6 months with a combination of anti-TB drugs; drug resistant TB is a particular problem with HIV patients.

❏ HIV and TB occurring together is a major public health problem worldwide.

❏ In patients with HIV the lung can be involved in infectious and noninfectious conditions; Kaposi's sarcoma and lymphomas of the lung are recognized malignant complications of HIV infection that can involve the lung.

RECOMMENDED READING

Pneumonia Guidelines Subcommittee, Standards of Care Committee of the British Thoracic Society (2001) Guidelines for the management of community acquire pneumonia. *Thorax* **56** (Suppl IV).

Chemotherapy and management of tuberculosis in the United Kingdom: recommendations 1998. *Thorax* 1998;**53**:536–48.

Control and prevention of tuberculosis in the United Kingdom: Code of practice 2000. *Thorax* 2000;**55**:887–901.

All the above guidelines and subsequent updates can be downloaded from the British Thoracic Society website (www.brit-thoracic.org.uk).

Chapter 11 Suppurative lung conditions

INTRODUCTION

This chapter encompasses three separate lung diseases not covered elsewhere in this book, namely bronchiectasis, cystic fibrosis, and lung abscess. Other infective conditions, such as pneumonia, tuberculosis, and opportunist lung infections, are covered in Chapter 10, and empyema is included in Chapter 9.

BRONCHIECTASIS

The word bronchiectasis is derived from the Greek meaning stretching or extension of the air pipes. Nowadays bronchiectasis is usually defined as a condition characterized by chronic dilatation of one or more bronchi. Bronchiectasis is a significant cause of morbidity and mortality around the world, but estimates of its frequency are hard to establish, largely because of difficulties in standardizing the diagnosis of the condition. Dilatation of the airways cannot be ascertained by clinical examination and nor can bronchiectasis be diagnosed from a plain chest radiograph.

In years gone by direct imaging of the airways by use of contrast media placed there was used to produce a 'bronchogram' (78). Nowadays, high resolution computerized tomography (HRCT) is the investigation of choice (79). As this is not available in some countries where bronchiectasis prevalence is likely to be high, the true burden of the condition is likely to be underestimated. The prevalence of bronchiectasis will also vary according to the prevalence of causative co-morbidities, which may vary considerably from country to country and with time; for example post-pertussis bronchiectasis will now be uncommon in western Europe.

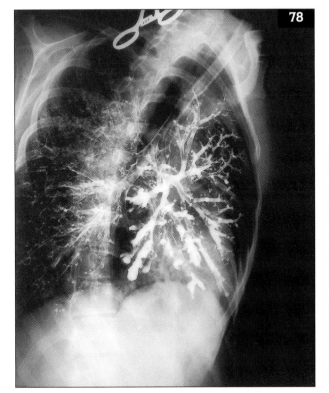

78 A 'bronchogram' showing saccular and fusiform bronchiectasis. Nowadays, a CT thorax would be used for diagnosing bronchiectasis rather than bronchography

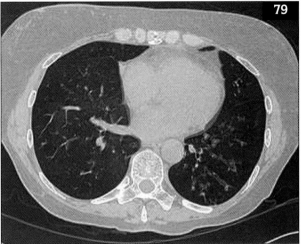

79 A CT thorax showing thickened airway walls and dilated airways; these are often best realized by visualizing an airway with a calibre in excess of that usually seen so peripherally

The causes of bronchiectasis are shown in *Table 56*. While childhood measles and whooping cough, and post-tuberculous damage, are major causes of bronchiectasis worldwide, they are less common in Western Europe. In the latter the presentation of a patient with probable bronchiectasis is more likely to involve a comprehensive structured investigation into the possibility of ciliary dyskinesia, hypogamma-globulinaenia, alpha-1-antitrypsin deficiency or bronchopulmonary aspergillosis. Homozygous alpha-1-antitrypsin deficiency is usually correctly thought of as a cause of premature emphysema, but about 10% of homozygotes present instead with bronchiectasis. It is also important to note that while evidence of bronchiectasis from CT scans is commonly reported in cases of diffuse parenchymal lung disease (traction bronchiectasis), this is very much a secondary phenomenon and the clinical picture is dominated by the interstitial process.

CLINICAL FEATURES

Characteristic symptoms of bronchiectasis are a chronic cough productive of copious quantities of sputum, which may be complicated by haemoptysis and pneumonia. Breathlessness may be a feature, depending upon the extent of the pulmonary damage. Finger clubbing may be present in cases of extensive bronchiectasis and coarse crackles are often audible over areas of bronchiectasis on auscultation. The dilatation of the airways and increased secretions lead to impaired clearance of secretions and stasis. This often leads to increased infection and a vicious cycle of purulence, leading to inflammation and further bronchial damage, which itself predisposes to increased sepsis. This vicious cycle needs to be broken by good bronchial toilet, which involves the patient being taught how to undertake forced expiratory techniques and postural drainage to clear the affected lobe or lobes. This may need to be combined with the use of regular bronchodilators and courses of appropriate antibiotics (but not continuous antibiotics).

INVESTIGATIONS AND DIAGNOSIS

Investigations which may be necessary in suspected cases of bronchiectasis are shown in *Table 57*.

Table 56 Causes of bronchiectasis

Congenital causes and congenital predispositions to bronchiectasis
- ❏ Kartagener's syndrome (situs inversus, rhinosinusitis, and bronchiectasis)
- ❏ Other types of ciliary dysfunction
- ❏ Cystic fibrosis
- ❏ Hypogammaglobulinaemia
- ❏ Bronchomalacia
- ❏ Homozygous alpha-1-antitrypsin deficiency

Acquired bronchiectasis
- ❏ Childhood pneumonia (whooping cough, measles, and so on)
- ❏ Foreign body inhalation
- ❏ Tuberculosis
- ❏ Suppurative pneumonia
- ❏ Bronchopulmonary aspergillosis (which characteristically gives proximal airway bronchiectasis)
- ❏ Bronchial obstruction secondary to adenomas and carcinomas
- ❏ Diseases causing extensive fibrosis, for example, connective tissue disorders such as rheumatoid arthritis
- ❏ Associated with inflammatory bowel disease

Table 57 Investigations in bronchiectasis

Blood tests
- ❏ White cell count
- ❏ Erythrocyte sedimentation rate and C-reactive protein
- ❏ Immunoglobulins
- ❏ *Aspergillus* precipitin test
- ❏ Rheumatoid factor
- ❏ Alpha-1-antitrypsin levels

Sputum
- ❏ Acid-fast bacillus
- ❏ Culture and sensitivity
- ❏ Eosinophil count

Imaging
- ❏ Chest radiograph
- ❏ CT sinus examination
- ❏ High-resolution thin section CT scan

Other investigations
- ❏ Fibre-optic bronchoscopy
- ❏ Sweat test
- ❏ *Aspergillus* skin test
- ❏ Semen analysis

CYSTIC FIBROSIS

Cystic fibrosis is inherited as an autosomal recessive disorder, and occurs in approximately 1 in 2,500 live white births. More than 90% of patients with cystic fibrosis will die of lung disease, but the prognosis has improved considerably over the last few decades. In 1976 the median survival in the UK was approximately 18 years but by the 1990s it had improved to 29 years. Most people born with cystic fibrosis today can expect to live into their third or fourth decades. At the present time in the UK there are as many adults with cystic fibrosis as children. Most were diagnosed in childhood having presented with meconium ileus, rectal prolapse, failure to thrive, or repeated chest infections.

Most mutations are associated with pancreatic insufficiency and the patient presents in childhood, but it is important to realize that a small number of patients have mutations associated with relatively normal pancreatic function. In these cases diagnosis can be delayed and patients may first present in adolescence or in early adult life with sinusitis, nasal polyps, or a chronic productive cough, or during investigations for infertility.

INVESTIGATIONS AND DIAGNOSIS

The diagnosis of cystic fibrosis is made by means of a sweat test. An abnormal result (chloride > 60 mmol/l) or a borderline test (chloride 40–60 mmol/l) should always be repeated. If positive the diagnosis is confirmed. If persistently borderline, genotyping for the most common mutations should be undertaken.

MANAGEMENT

Treatment of the disorder is currently symptomatic and prevention of (further) pulmonary damage is the main aim. In children *Staphylococcus aureus* is the main pathogen; in adolescents and adults it is *Pseudomonas aeruginosa*. Repeated courses of high-dose intravenous antibiotics are needed in older patients, but regular nebulized antibiotics (tobramycin, colistin or gentamycin) may also have a beneficial effect, perhaps by increasing the interval between exacerbations. Trials of inhaled steroids are also indicated, as is the symptomatic use of bronchodilators. Nebulized recombinant human DNase can reduce sputum viscosity, improve lung function, and reduce exacerbations, but should only be instituted regularly after the demonstration of an objective benefit.

COMPLICATIONS

Complications of cystic fibrosis include diabetes, biliary cirrhosis, pulmonary heart disease, pneumothorax, and infertility in males and reduced fertility in females. Heart–lung transplantation and, on occasion, lung, liver, and pancreas transplantation can achieve excellent results.

LUNG ABSCESS

A lung abscess is a suppurative lung infection associated with the death of lung tissue in the centre of an area of infection. It is commonly visualized as a cavitating opacity on imaging (80). See *Table 58* for its causes.

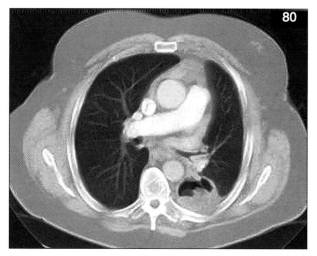

80 A posteriorly placed abscess in the left lung

Table 58 Causes of lung abscess

❑ Aspiration of infective organisms from the upper airways

❑ Bronchial obstruction secondary to tumour or foreign body with distal infection, infarction, and lung cavitation

❑ Blood-borne infection – septicaemia associated with hospitalization or IV drug abuse

❑ Spread of infection from below the diaphragm

❑ A complication of pneumonia

❑ Pulmonary embolism and infarction with subsequent infection of infarcted lung

DIFFERENTIAL DIAGNOSIS

Other diseases not primarily due to infection may mimic a lung abscess or be confused with a lung abscess. These include:

- Cavitating carcinoma. The usual situation is that a solid tumour mass has outstripped its blood supply with the centre of the tumour then dying and the contents being expectorated.
- Pulmonary infarct. Pulmonary infarcts may cavitate. While pulmonary infarction in the upper lobe is less usual than infarction elsewhere in the lung, infarcts in this area may be more likely than elsewhere to cavitate, reflecting death of the tissue. This may occur with or without associated infection.
- Pulmonary TB (see Chapter 10, page 113). This may be associated with cavitation in the apicoposterior segments of the upper lobe, or in the apical segments of the lower lobes. It may occasionally be confused with a nontuberculous lung abscess.
- Infection within a bulla. Large air-filled sacs, occurring within or without the context of associated emphysema, are aerated but often not ventilated. Infection reaching these bullae may cause an inflammatory response, which leads to secretions within the bullae which cannot easily be drained. This may mimic a lung abscess.
- Wegener's granulomatosis may be associated with the death of lung tissue and cavitation.
- Hiatus hernia. It is very important to remember that entry of a portion of gas-filled stomach into the chest may be mistaken for a lung abscess. The location of the 'abscess' behind the heart shadow (**81**) is a clue to the correct diagnosis of a hiatus hernia.

Most lung abscesses reflect the migration of commensal organisms in the oropharynx into the lung. This probably happens in all of us on a regular basis, but an intact immune system, coughing, and an effective mucociliary escalator prevent such a scenario from progressing to infection and lung abscess formation in most of us for most of the time. Lung abscess formation is more likely to occur if the number of organisms in the orophranyx increases, or if there is impairment of defence mechanisms.

Any of the following will enhance the risk of lung abscess:

- Dental sepsis.
- Sinus disease.
- Neurological disease affecting pharynx, larynx or oesophagus.
- Obstruction in the larynx (e.g. by tumour) or oesophagus (e.g. achalasia, tumour or hiatus hernia) or presence of a pharyngeal pouch.
- Impaired consciousness secondary to sleep, alcohol or drug abuse, general anaesthesia or epilepsy.

CAUSATIVE ORGANISMS IN LUNG ABSCESSES

The aspiration of organisms from the oropharynx usually involves aspiration of multiple organisms, usually anaerobes. Aspiration occurring in hospitalized patients may lead to lung abscess formation associated with Gram-negative bacteria and staphylococci. Pneumonia that cavitates or is associated with abscess formation may be due to *Mycobacterium tuberculosis*, *Staphylococcus aureus* or *Klebsiella pneumonia*. Blood-borne infections, especially *Staphylococcus aureus*, can result in single or multiple lung abscess formation, which is more likely in IV drug abusers or hospitalized patients who may have had repeated intravenous lines. Occasionally hepatic abscesses, such as an amoebic abscess, may spread through the diaphragm and lead to lung abscess formation.

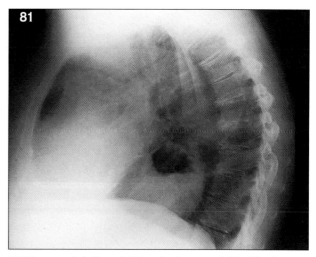

81 The rounded air-containing shadow seen behind the heart shadow is a hiatus hernia; its position should help avoid confusion with a lung abscess

CLINICAL FEATURES

Patients present complaining of high fever, usually of relatively sudden onset, accompanied by cough, profound malaise, and pleuritic pain. They may produce purulent blood-stained sputum and they look unwell and toxic. There may or may not be focal signs to elicit in the chest and, depending on the length of the history, they may have lost a considerable amount of weight and may develop finger clubbing. If the abscess is close to the visceral pleura they may develop a complicating empyema and have dullness to percussion on clinical examination.

INVESTIGATIONS AND DIAGNOSIS

The diagnosis is made radiographically but it is important to consider the differential diagnosis and to be aware that lung cancer, pulmonary infarction, and Wegener's granulomotosis, for example, may all mimic a lung abscess. Samples should be sent for microbiological examination, clearly alerting the microbiologist to the clinical scenario so that anaerobic organisms, TB, and less common organisms – such as *Actinomyces* and *Nocardia* – may all be looked for.

MANAGEMENT

Antibiotics should be started pending the results of the microbiological investigations, and a suitable regimen would be high-dose penicillin, often plus metronidazole or, if there are multiple abscesses in an IV drug abuser or someone who has recently been hospitalized, antistaphylococcal treatment should be added.

Physiotherapy is essential. Bronchoscopy is often necessary to exclude bronchial obstruction. Patients with large abscesses need to be carefully observed, for occasionally rupture of the abscess into the bronchial tree can lead to extensive flooding of the rest of the lung with necrotic inflammatory material. If intensive prolonged physiotherapy does not lead to satisfactory removal of the abscess contents, then percutaneous drainage or even, occasionally, surgical resection of the abscess is needed.

Chapter 12 Sleep-related breathing disorders

INTRODUCTION

Sleep is important. Animals deprived of sleep die but the function of sleep remains a mystery. The state of sleep interacts with breathing in a number of important ways. For example, respiratory drive alters which, in susceptible patients, may cause nocturnal hypoventilation or central sleep apnoea (cessation of breathing due to loss of respiratory drive). This chapter focuses on one of the commonest sleep-related breathing disorders, obstructive sleep apnoea.

OBSTRUCTIVE SLEEP APNOEA

Obstructive sleep apnoea is neither a new disease nor a rare disease but it has only recently become widely recognized. It is surprising that this disease went unnoticed for so long, especially if one visits a sleep clinic and listens carefully to patients with obstructive sleep apnoea and their bed partners! Embarrassingly for doctors, in the 1830s Charles Dickens appears to have described the condition in *The Pickwick Papers*. His fat boy, Joe, was an extremely loud snorer and so sleepy that he even nodded off during meals.

AETIOLOGY AND PATHOPHYSIOLOGY

Obstructive sleep apnoea occurs as a result of obstruction of the upper airway during sleep. Very occasionally there is an obvious cause, such as very large tonsils, but, more usually, the exact mechanism and site of obstruction are obscure. The problem seems to stem from the dual function of the pharynx, which needs to propel food down into the oesophagus as well as act as an airway. From an engineering point of view, an airway ideally needs to be splinted open like the 'elephant tubing' of a vacuum cleaner. In the trachea this function is carried out by the cartilaginous tracheal rings. On the other hand propelling food requires peristalsis and a floppy structure capable of constriction, like the oesophagus. To function as an airway the pharynx needs to be held open during inspiration, when the pressure inside will fall. The way in which this is achieved is complicated and involves various muscles. Some of the muscular actions can be demonstrated as follows: if the mouth is closed, the nose held, and the person sniffs, negative pressure is generated in the pharynx. If the same action is repeated with a finger and thumb on the hyoid bone, the forward movement of the hyoid bone, as a result of contraction of the glenohyoid

muscle, can be felt. This movement increases the size of the upper airway. It is muscular actions such as this which maintain the patency of the upper airway.

In obstructive sleep apnoea the mechanisms for keeping the upper airway open fail and the airway becomes occluded. During sleep, particularly rapid eye movement sleep, there is a decrease in muscle tone. As the muscles which maintain the patency of the upper airway relax, the upper airway may obstruct. Respiratory movements continue but there is no airflow. Eventually the patient will tend to wake up and, as this happens, muscular tone returns, the airway opens and breathing starts again, often with a loud snort. The patient then falls back to sleep and the cycle recurs. As a result, sleep is fragmented and the patient wakes unrefreshed and feels sleepy in the day.

CLINICAL FEATURES

Obstructive sleep apnoea may affect children or the elderly but prevalence reaches a peak in the fifth and sixth decades. There is an association with obesity. It is a common condition affecting perhaps 5% of middle-aged men, though women are less often affected. The clinical features are listed in *Table 59*.

Most patients snore. Snoring is typically extremely loud and easily heard in another part of the house. Snoring of this severity may be very damaging to relationships but is not necessarily accompanied by

---

Table 59 Clinical features of obstructive sleep apnoea

- ❑ Loud snoring
- ❑ Witnessed apnoeas often terminating with a snort
- ❑ Nocturnal choking
- ❑ Unrefreshing sleep
- ❑ Daytime somnolence
- ❑ Nocturia
- ❑ Night sweats
- ❑ Decreased libido

obstructive apnoeas. When it is, the resulting sleep fragmentation can cause unrefreshing sleep and daytime sleepiness. Bed partners witness apnoeas, sometimes ending with a snort, and occasionally patients themselves are aware of this, or associated choking episodes. Nocturia, night sweats, and impotence may also be features. Sometimes the symptoms follow an increase in weight and many patients are known hypertensives. Not infrequently there is a history of loud snoring or sleep apnoea in the family. Bed partners often report that snoring and apnoeas are worse after alcohol.

On examination there may be no obvious structural cause predisposing to obstructive apnoea, though many patients are obese with fat necks, and some have retrognathia. Examination of the mouth may reveal a large tongue. Sometimes the soft palate is long and the uvula out of view behind the tongue. It may be apparent that space at the back of the throat is restricted. Frequently, as a result of snoring, the uvula is red and oedematous. A variety of problems within the nose may cause nasal obstruction which may contribute to the problem by lowering the inspiratory pharyngeal pressure. Some of the factors which predispose to the development of obstructive sleep apnoea are listed in *Table 60*.

It is important to realize that there are many other causes of sleepiness (*Table 61*).

Table 60 Predisposing factors for obstructive sleep apnoea

❏ Obesity (collar size > 17 inches [43 cm])

❏ Retrognathia

❏ Nasal obstruction

❏ Hypnotics and alcohol

❏ Neurological disorders

❏ Renal failure

❏ Acromegaly

❏ Hypothyroidism

Table 61 Other causes of excessive sleepiness

❏ Not enough time allocated to sleep

❏ Circardian rhythm disturbance:

    Shift work

    Jet lag

    Phase alteration syndromes (sleepiness out of phase with night)

❏ Narcolepsy

❏ Idiopathic hypersomnolence

❏ Periodic limb movement disorder

❏ Drugs and alcohol

❏ Depressive illness

INVESTIGATIONS AND DIAGNOSIS

To confirm the diagnosis of obstructive sleep apnoea, it is usual to perform a sleep study, ideally at home, where patients are likely to sleep best. Various technologies to do this have been developed. For example sensors can be attached to detect airflow at the nose and mouth, snoring, thoracic and abdominal respiratory movements, pulse rate, and arterial oxygen saturation (82). If the airflow stops and the respiratory movements continue this implies an obstructive apnoea (as opposed to a central apnoea when there is no drive to breathe). This may be followed by desaturation and a rise in pulse rate associated with arousal when breathing restarts. In practice reliably detecting respiratory movements in the obese can be difficult and, in a typical case, a diagnosis can often be made without the full range of measurements.

A sleep study is also useful to obtain some index of the severity of the condition. The number of apnoeic events per hour provides some measure of this but it is important to remember that, without an electro-encephalogram, it is not possible to be sure that the patient is asleep when the measurements are being made and this could lead to an underestimate of severity.

MANAGEMENT

Patients with sleep apnoea are more likely to have accidents while driving and should be advised of their duty to avoid putting others at risk. In patients who are obese the first line of treatment should be weight reduction. In practice this is difficult to achieve, and symptomatic obstructive sleep apnoea may remain a problem even in those who lose weight. All patients with abnormal sleepiness should be advised to allow adequate time for sleep and to keep to a regular sleep–wake pattern ('sleep hygiene'). Other general measures include reduction of excessive alcohol consumption, especially in the evenings, and avoidance of sleeping tablets. In occasional, usually mildly affected, patients, apnoeic episodes only occur in the supine position and it may be possible to train the patient to sleep on his side (perhaps with the help of a ball sewn into the back of the night clothes).

Measures to maintain the patency of the pharynx will prevent obstructive apnoea and the associated arousals and sleep fragmentation. Advancing the mandible with a splint increases the space behind the tongue and may be effective if this is the site of the obstruction, especially if there is retrognathia. Whatever the site of the obstruction, increasing the pressure within the upper airway will tend to prevent airway collapse but this requires continuous positive airway pressure (CPAP), usually administered via a nasal mask attached to a pump (83). In general patients will not persevere with these treatments unless they derive considerable symptomatic benefit, but, for those with excessive daytime sleepiness, improvements are often dramatic and the patient's life may be transformed.

Various operations have been devised with the

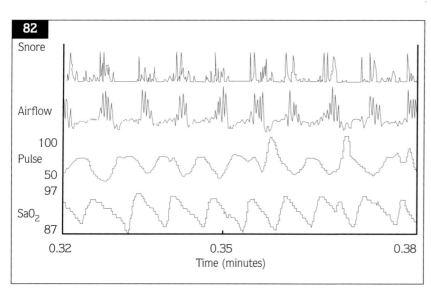

82 A printout from a home sleep study performed on a patient with obstructive sleep apnoea. The top channel shows snoring measured with a microphone (arbitrary units). Airflow measured at the mouth and nose with a thermistor is below (arbitrary units). The bottom two traces are pulse rate and oxygen saturation, both measured with a pulse oximeter. Notice the cyclical snoring, which coincides with airflow. When the airway obstructs both the airflow and snoring cease. After a lag the oxygen saturation falls and the pulse rate rises as the patient is aroused. As his sleep state lightens the muscles in the pharynx open the airway and the breathing and snoring start again. This happens repeatedly, sleep is fragmented, and daytime somnolence results

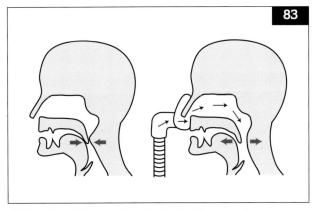

83 Sleeping with a nasal mask which delivers continuous positive airway pressure prevents occlusion of the upper airway. Arousals are prevented, sleep quality is improved and the patient feels more refreshed in the morning

aim of eliminating the obstruction that is the root cause of the problem. While individual patients may benefit from jaw advancement in cases of severe retrognathia, or from tonsillectomy, results have generally been disappointing.

OBESITY HYPOVENTILATION SYNDROME

Extremely obese patients may hypoventilate when asleep and sometimes also during the day when the daytime arterial PCO_2 is raised. They may complain of headaches, especially in the morning. Sometimes there is associated right heart failure. A proportion of these patients have obstructive sleep apnoea and may respond to nasal CPAP but some need nocturnal noninvasive ventilation.

NATURAL HISTORY AND PROGNOSIS

Many patients with obstructive sleep apnoea, especially those with severe sleepiness, benefit greatly from treatment with nocturnal nasal CPAP. In the UK the licensing authority may permit patients who have been successfully treated to hold a driving licence. But the treatment is not without its difficulties and much depends on the initial support given when CPAP is started. Some patients remain sleepy despite optimal treatment. It is important to advise all patients on sleep hygiene and to exclude other causes of somnolence. Patients with residual sleepiness may benefit from the wakefulness-promoting drug, modafinil.

SUMMARY
- Obstructive sleep apnoea is common, affecting up to 5% of middle-aged men.
- Loud snoring and excessive daytime sleepiness are key features.
- Drivers with untreated obstructive sleep apnoea are more likely to have a crash.
- Treatment with nocturnal nasal CPAP can be very effective.

RECOMMENDED READING

Sheerson JM *Sleep Medicine: A Guide to Sleep and its Disorders*. 2005 Blackwell Science Ltd, Oxford.

Douglas NJ *Clinicians' Guide to Sleep Medicine*. 2002 Arnold, London.

Scottish Intercollegiate Guidelines Network (SIGN). Management of obstructive sleep apnoea/hypopnea syndrome in adults; a National Clinical Guideline. www.sign.ac.uk

ACKNOWLEDGEMENTS

83 Adapted from a drawing by Hugh Cummin.

Chapter 13 Respiratory failure

INTRODUCTION

Respiratory failure is defined as a condition characterized by failure to maintain an arterial oxygen tension of greater than 8 kPa while breathing room air. The failure to maintain a PaO_2 of 8 kPa (hypoxaemia) may be associated with a normal or low (type I respiratory failure) or elevated (> 6 kPa) (type II respiratory failure) arterial tension of carbon dioxide.

AETIOLOGY AND PATHOPHYSIOLOGY

The two processes that are central to the maintenance of normal arterial tensions of oxygen and carbon dioxide are (a) the ventilatory muscle pump mechanism that is responsible for the movement of air to and from the gas exchanging surface of the lungs and (b) the process of gas exchange at the level of the alveoli (movement of oxygen into the pulmonary arterial blood and carbon dioxide into the atmosphere), which in turn is predicated on the presence of sufficient surface area of gas-exchanging tissue matched by an adequate pulmonary blood flow (ventilation–perfusion match). A disruption of any one of these related processes can result in failure to maintain normal arterial tensions of oxygen and carbon dioxide.

The various conditions listed usually affect predominantly one of these two processes; diseases affecting the ventilatory pump mechanism mainly result in type II (hypercapnic) respiratory failure while conditions causing a ventilation–perfusion mismatch due to loss of gas-exchanging surface result in type I (hypoxaemic only) respiratory failure (84).

CLINICAL FEATURES

It is important to bear in mind that while the clinical features may help establish the cause of respiratory failure, the diagnosis itself rests on the measurement of arterial blood gases.

HISTORY

There are no symptoms characteristic of respiratory failure; the symptoms are essentially those of the underlying cause. Although conditions causing respiratory failure present with symptoms referable to the

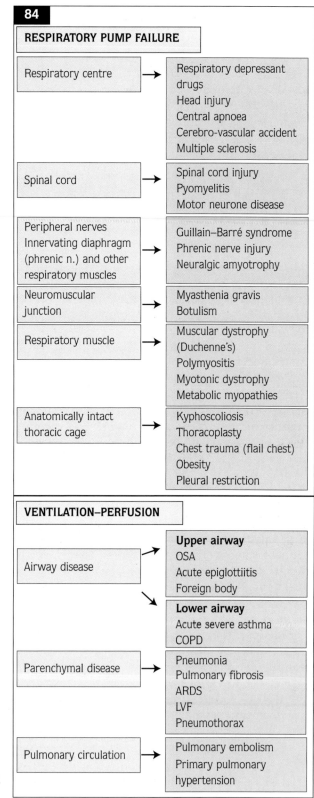

84

RESPIRATORY PUMP FAILURE

Respiratory centre	→	Respiratory depressant drugs Head injury Central apnoea Cerebro-vascular accident Multiple sclerosis
Spinal cord	→	Spinal cord injury Pyomyelitis Motor neurone disease
Peripheral nerves Innervating diaphragm (phrenic n.) and other respiratory muscles	→	Guillain–Barré syndrome Phrenic nerve injury Neuralgic amyotrophy
Neuromuscular junction	→	Myasthenia gravis Botulism
Respiratory muscle	→	Muscular dystrophy (Duchenne's) Polymyositis Myotonic dystrophy Metabolic myopathies
Anatomically intact thoracic cage	→	Kyphoscoliosis Thoracoplasty Chest trauma (flail chest) Obesity Pleural restriction

VENTILATION–PERFUSION

Airway disease	↗	**Upper airway** OSA Acute epiglottiitis Foreign body
	↘	**Lower airway** Acute severe asthma COPD
Parenchymal disease	→	Pneumonia Pulmonary fibrosis ARDS LVF Pneumothorax
Pulmonary circulation	→	Pulmonary embolism Primary pulmonary hypertension

84 Ventilatory pump mechanism and ventilation–perfusion mismatch in respiratory failure. ARDS, acute respiratory distress syndrome; COPD, chronic obstructive pulmonary disease; LVF, left ventricular failure; OSAS, obstructive sleep apnoea

respiratory system (breathlessness, wheeze, and so on) some, particularly those causing insidious type II failure in the context of immobility or effort intolerance (e.g. respiratory muscle weakness associated with neurological conditions – Guillain–Barré syndrome, motor neurone disease, multiple sclerosis), may offer no symptoms referable to the respiratory system, and the condition has to be actively sought. Some patients with type II respiratory failure may complain of a throbbing morning headache, reflecting nocturnal worsening of respiratory failure and carbon dioxide-induced cerebral vasodilation.

The rate of onset of the condition may provide some clues as to the aetiology (85). It must however be borne in mind that some conditions, particularly neuromuscular disorders, show a variable tendency to progression and may present in chronic rather than subacute fashion. While most conditions cause type I or II respiratory failure exclusively, the picture may be complicated by the presence of more than one disease, e.g. acute pneumonia occurring in the context of stable type II failure due to COPD or kyphoscoliosis may present with type II rather than type I failure.

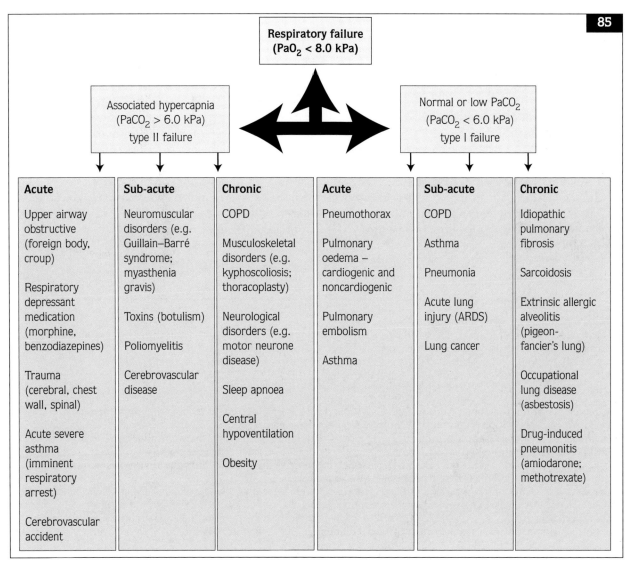

85 Causes of respiratory failure depending on the mode of onset (acute, minutes to hours; sub-acute, days to weeks; chronic, months to years). NB: Categories are not mutually exclusive. ARDS, acute respiratory distress syndrome; COPD, chronic obstructive pulmonary disease

PHYSICAL EXAMINATION

Cyanosis is traditionally described as a feature of hypoxaemia and must be looked for, but it is not a reliable indicator of either the presence or severity of respiratory failure. The respiratory rate may be increased or decreased. The features of hypercapnia may be evident (bounding pulse, warm peripheries, tremor or flap), as may signs of cor pulmonale. Orthopnoea is commonly a feature of left ventricular failure, but can occasionally be the presenting feature of diaphragmatic weakness. Paradoxical abdominal wall movement (drawing in during inspiration and distension on expiration) is also a feature of diaphragmatic weakness. Chest wall abnormalities (kyphoscoliosis, thoraco-plasty, and flail chest post-trauma) must be examined for. The findings on examination of the lung fields are dictated by the underlying condition causing respiratory failure (COPD, interstitial lung disease, neurological illness, and so on). Carbon dioxide retention can cause papilloedema.

INVESTIGATIONS AND DIAGNOSIS

ARTERIAL BLOOD GAS ANALYSIS

Arterial blood gas analysis is central to the diagnosis of respiratory failure for the following reasons:

❑ Measurements of arterial oxygen and carbon dioxide tensions are essential for the diagnosis of respiratory failure ($PaO_2 < 8kPa$) and the classification of it as type I or II, indicating possible causes (85).

❑ The arterial pH and bicarbonate levels are a useful guide to the urgency with which respiratory support needs to be established. Chronic hypercapnia (as happens with respiratory muscle weakness or stable COPD) is associated with the body's homeostatic mechanisms preventing acidosis and maintaining pH by retaining bicarbonate. The presence of acidosis (pH < 7.3) in such illnesses indicates a state of decompensation and warrants immediate consideration of respiratory support (see below).

❑ It helps in the calculation of the alveolar–arterial oxygen gradient, which provides some clues as to the cause of respiratory failure and is a more sensitive indicator of the disruption of gas exchange than arterial gas tensions alone in type I respiratory failure (Box 6).

PULSE OXIMETRY

Oxygen saturations can be measured by pulse oximetry and, particularly in type I respiratory failure, can be a guide to the severity of the condition and response to treatment. It is important to bear in mind that pulse oximetry *does not* give any indication of carbon dioxide levels and is to be used with caution in monitoring type II respiratory failure, especially when supplemental oxygen is given. Severe carbon dioxide retention can exist in a patient with normal oxygen saturations.

BOX 6 The alveolar–arterial oxygen gradient

The alveolar–arterial oxygen gradient is the difference between the tensions of oxygen in the alveolus and the arterial circulation. It is normally < 3 kPa and increases with age to around 4 kPa at age 80.
It is calculated thus:

$$PAO_2 - PaO_2 = \left(FIO_2 - \frac{PaCO_2}{0.8} \right) - PaO_2$$

In general, conditions causing type II respiratory failure due to ventilatory pump failure (respiratory muscle weakness, respiratory depression due to central causes) are associated with hypoxia and preserved $A{-}aO_2$ gradient.
Example: A patient with motor neurone disease presents with type II respiratory failure, with a PaO_2 of 8 kPa and a $PaCO_2$ of 8 kPa, breathing room air. The $A{-}aO_2$ gradient is: (21 – 8 / 0.8) – 8 = (21 – 10) – 8 = 3 kPa
Occasionally the $A{-}aO_2$ gradient is elevated even when the arterial O_2 and CO_2 tensions are not in the respiratory failure range, indicating the presence of deranged gas exchange.
Example: A 23 year-old female on the oral contraceptive pill presents after a long aeroplane flight with pleuritic chest pain. Arterial blood gas analysis breathing room air shows a PaO_2 of 9.2 kPa and a $PaCO_2$ of 4 kPa.
$A{-}aO_2$ gradient = (21 – 4 / 0.8) – 9.2 = (21 – 5) – 9.2 = 6.8 kPa (raised), suggesting the possibility of pulmonary embolism, although $PaO2$ is greater than the usual defining level of respiratory failure.

FIO_2, fractional inspired oxygen concentration; PAO_2, alveolar oxygen; $PaCO_2$, arterial carbon dioxide; PaO_2, arterial oxygen

LUNG FUNCTION TESTS

These are of value in diagnosing the disease causing respiratory failure but are seldom performed in patients acutely ill with respiratory failure. An exception is in patients with incipient respiratory muscle weakness due to Guillain–Barré syndrome, where serial measurements of vital capacity are crucial in anticipating respiratory failure and the need for respiratory support.

Conditions like COPD, asthma, and interstitial lung disease exhibit characteristic patterns of abnormality on spirometry, lung volume, and diffusing capacity measurements.

The diaphragm is the main respiratory muscle and its weakness can cause respiratory failure. Diaphragmatic weakness (except post-traumatic, including iatrogenic) is of insidious onset and gradual progression. Exclusive weakness of the intercostals and other respiratory muscles causing respiratory failure is virtually unknown, while weakness of one hemidiaphragm seldom causes respiratory failure.

Diseases causing respiratory muscle weakness are also associated with a typical constellation of abnormalities, the most important of which is a fall in VC of > 20% on adoption of the supine posture. Orthopnoea and paradoxical abdominal wall movement are important clinical features; decreased maximal inspiratory and expiratory pressures (P_I and P_E max) measured at the mouth are other features.

IMAGING

A chest radiograph may show features of the underlying disease (pneumonia, pulmonary oedema – cardiogenic [enlarged heart] or noncardiogenic [normal-sized heart], pneumothorax, pulmonary fibrosis, and so on).

Severe respiratory failure with clear lung fields should raise the suspicion of:

❑ Pulmonary thromboembolic or vascular disease (type I failure) (relevant imaging techniques here are a VQ scan, spiral CT scan, and pulmonary angiography).

❑ The various diseases associated with a failure of the ventilatory pump (lung fields, although clear, are apt to be small owing to the elevated position of the paralysed or weak diaphragm).

OTHER INVESTIGATIONS

Phrenic nerve conduction studies and diaphragmatic electromyography (EMG) recordings are of value in diaphragmatic weakness, enabling detection of the level of the lesion (nerve, neuromuscular junction or muscle).

MANAGEMENT

Aims of treatment:

❑ Prevention of life-threatening hypoxia.

❑ Prevention of life-threatening hypercapnia.

❑ Management of the underlying cause of the respiratory failure.

Oxygen therapy

Oxygen therapy is dealt with in detail in Chapter 8. The following general principles apply in the use of oxygen therapy for respiratory failure:

❑ In the management of type I respiratory failure, where there is no danger of supplemental oxygen worsening hypercapnia, the highest fraction of inspired oxygen required to achieve satisfactory tissue oxygenation (as reflected by an SaO_2 of > 92%) should be used. In cases of type II respiratory failure, particularly in acute exacerbations of COPD, where there is a danger of uncontrolled oxygen therapy worsening hypercapnia, the minimum FIO_2 required to keep oxygen saturations over 90% should be used.

❑ Failure of high fractions of supplemental oxygen alone to improve oxygenation must prompt early consideration of ventilatory support (see below).

❑ When blood gas analysis is performed on a patient on oxygen therapy, the fraction of inspired oxygen must be carefully noted before conclusions are drawn.

❑ Oxygen at high flow rates can irritate the upper airway mucosa and this tendency is reduced by humidification.

❑ Oxygen toxicity is a well recognized, if rare, problem in infants and children in whom high concentrations (60–100%) have been used for long periods of time; there is little reason to avoid its use in the short term (24 hours) in adults in acute respiratory failure.

Management of hypercapnia

While hypoxia can often be managed by increasing the fraction of inspired oxygen, hypercapnia requires an improved efficacy of the ventilatory pump. In the setting of acute respiratory failure this is best provided by either partially or totally supporting the patient's respiratory effort with mechanical devices. The widespread availability of these devices, in particular the advent of noninvasive ventilation techniques, has diminished considerably the role of respiratory stimulant drugs like doxapram. Mechanical ventilatory support can be provided by:

❏ Positive pressure ventilation, where the device inflates the lungs by the application of positive pressure into the airways, either noninvasively by a tight-fitting nasal or facial mask (86) or invasively via a tube in the trachea.

❏ Negative pressure ventilation, where the lungs are inflated by negative pressure applied to the chest or abdominal wall (cuirass or tank ventilators).

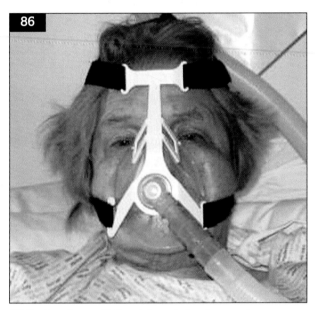

86 Noninvasive ventilation delivered via a face mask

Negative pressure ventilators are not widely used.

In addition to improving the elimination of carbon dioxide, ventilatory support also affords the fatigued respiratory muscles some rest, expediting their return to normal. In general the following warrant consideration of ventilatory support:

❏ Progressive hypercapnia with acidosis (pH < 7.3).

❏ Hypoxia refractory to increasing fractional inspired oxygen concentration (FIO_2).

❏ Profound exhaustion in the context of severe tachypnoea and respiratory distress (respiratory rate of > 30/min).

❏ Altered states of consciousness, including restlessness and coma attributable to respiratory failure.

The decision to employ an invasive or noninvasive technique of ventilation is dictated by the clinical circumstances (*Table 62*). It is important to note that with both noninvasive and invasive techniques, supplementary oxygen therapy can be provided, although the scope for this is limited with noninvasive techniques.

DOMICILIARY VENTILATION

In patients with chronic respiratory failure, particularly due to kyphoscoliosis, thoracoplasty, and neuromuscular disorders, assisted ventilation is carried out in the home setting in the long term. Usually, noninvasive techniques are used and, if possible, respiratory support is provided during the

Table 62 Features of invasive and noninvasive ventilation

	Noninvasive ventilation (NIV)	Invasive positive pressure ventilation
Principle	Respiratory support delivered through a tight fitting nasal or facial mask	Respiratory support delivered through an endotracheal tube
Advantages	Noninvasive No need for sedation or paralysis Patient awake; able to eat, drink, and communicate Can be delivered in a ward setting	Complete control of the airway No concern about patient cooperation
Contraindications	Unconscious or uncooperative patient (absolute) Bulbar weakness (absolute) Copious secretions (relative)	None unless there is a specific advance directive from the patient forbidding its use
Limitations	Patient must be conscious and cooperative No control of airways Tracheobronchila toilet not facilitated May induce claustrophobia	Need for sedation and paralysis Weaning may pose ethical difficulties Can be delivered only in the intensive care setting

night only, thus limiting the adverse impact of the treatment on day-to-day activities.

Advance directives

In most cases of acute respiratory failure the decision to institute ventilatory support is made by the professionals involved without any explicit involvement of the patient. However, in some instances, particularly in patients in whom the episode is a worsening of a long-term condition with a tendency to terminal decline (motor neurone disease, COPD), the decision to intubate and ventilate may be dictated by the previously expressed wishes of the patient, legally expressed in the form of an advance directive ('living will'). When formulated under due processes of law such documents are binding.

MANAGEMENT OF THE UNDERLYING CAUSE OF RESPIRATORY FAILURE

While supplementary oxygen therapy and mechanical ventilatory assistance stabilize the respiratory status of the patient, treatment of the underlying condition must be given equal consideration in the management of acute respiratory failure (e.g. naloxone for narcotic-induced respiratory failure, antibiotics for pneumonia, steroids and bronchodilators for asthma and COPD, intercostal tube drainage for pneumo-thorax, and so on). In certain conditions supplemental oxygen therapy and ventilatory support may be part of the long-term management of the underlying cause of the failure.

SUMMARY

- ❑ Respiratory failure is defined as the inability to maintain an arterial oxygen tension of > 8 kPa breathing room air. Carbon dioxide tensions may be normal or low (type I respiratory failure) or elevated (> 6.0 kPa; type II respiratory failure).
- ❑ Respiratory failure can result from malfunction of the ventilatory pump mechanism (respiratory centre, neuromuscular connections, and thoracic cage apparatus) and/or a mismatch between alveolar ventilation and perfusion (VQ mismatch).
- ❑ Arterial blood gas analysis is central to the diagnosis of respiratory failure and its management.
- ❑ A full history, physical examination, and investigations (including lung function tests and imaging techniques) usually enable a specific cause for the condition to be identified.
- ❑ Supplemental oxygen therapy and ventilatory support are the main modalities used to treat respiratory failure while investigations are in progress and the underlying disease is managed.
- ❑ Ventilatory support can be provided invasively via an endotracheal tube or noninvasively via a tight-fitting nasal or face mask.

Chapter 14 Pulmonary vascular problems

INTRODUCTION

Pulmonary emboli, pulmonary oedema, and secondary pulmonary hypertension are common problems for the clinician. Other pulmonary vascular disorders discussed in this chapter belong within the category of rare pulmonary diseases, but are important in clinical practice.

Before discussing these disorders, it is helpful to recall the structure and function of the normal pulmonary circulation (87). In addition to the pulmonary circulation, the lung also receives a systemic arterial supply via the bronchial arteries, which arise from the thoracic aorta. In each cardiac cycle the pulmonary circulation receives the entire cardiac output from the right ventricle via a branching system of arteries, arterioles then capillaries, before blood is returned to the left atrium through draining pulmonary veins. The meshwork of pulmonary capillaries delivers deoxygenated blood to the alveolar–capillary interface for gas exchange. The capillary bed also serves as a filtration unit for particulate material, and metabolizes important blood-borne chemicals.

PULMONARY VASCULAR PRESSURES

The pulmonary vascular bed operates as a low pressure, low resistance, highly compliant system. Low driving pulmonary artery pressures are possible since the lung apices are approximately 15 cm vertically above the heart. As a result, normal pulmonary arteries have thinner walls and less smooth muscle than their systemic counterparts, and the pulmonary artery and right ventricular pressures are normally substantially lower than aortic and left ventricular pressures.

$$\text{Blood flow*} = \frac{\text{driving pressure head}}{\text{resistance to flow}} = \frac{\text{pulmonary arterial} - \text{pulmonary venous pressure}}{\text{pulmonary vascular resistance}}$$

* Blood flow = cardiac output

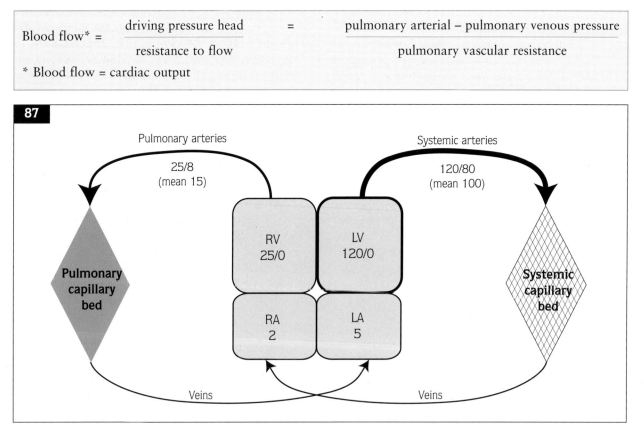

87 Comparison of pulmonary and systemic circulations. Note the right-sided circular has lower ventricular and arterial pressures, thinner arterial walls, and a mesh-like capillary bed. All pressures in mmHg. LA, left atrium; LV, left ventricle; RA, right atrium; RV, right ventricle

The spare capacity of the pulmonary vascular bed

Under normal circumstances the pulmonary vascular bed has an extensive spare capacity since blood flow is unevenly distributed; at rest many areas of the lung are underperfused (particularly in the upper lobes owing to gravity). The spare capacity is crucial in three major settings:

❏ 'Matching' of pulmonary ventilation and perfusion. If alveoli in areas of the lung are unventilated for whatever reason (physiological or disease), perfusion to the alveoli is reduced to match. This is regulated by the process of hypoxic vasoconstriction: if the alveolar oxygen tension falls, local pulmonary arteries < 1,000 μm in diameter are actively vasoconstricted to divert blood flow to aerated regions of the lung.

❏ Maintaining a low pulmonary artery pressure if cardiac output is increased (e.g. exercise, pyrexia). If cardiac output is increased, the increased pulmonary blood flow is accommodated by increasing the cross section of the capillary bed by recruitment of additional capillaries from underperfused areas of the lung. This reduces the pulmonary vascular resistance and means that the pulmonary artery pressure can remain low.

❏ Maintaining a low pulmonary artery pressure if areas of the pulmonary vascular bed are lost (e.g. pulmonary emboli, parenchymal destruction in emphysema). Pulmonary artery pressure need not increase, even when up to 40–50% of the pulmonary vascular bed is obliterated. However, if pathology persists, the compensatory mechanisms are overwhelmed.

PULMONARY EMBOLI

Pulmonary emboli (PEs) account for approximately 1% of all admissions to general hospitals and are particularly prevalent in post-operative patients. The overwhelming majority are pulmonary thrombo-emboli, due to detached thrombin clots. These usually originate in deep venous thromboses (DVTs) of the legs or pelvic veins, though thromboemboli may also originate within the right-sided cardiac chambers. Nonthrombotic PEs include air, bulky tumour, fat, placental, amniotic fluid, parasitic, and septic emboli. Small microemboli are routinely cleared from the circulation. Larger or multiple emboli obstruct sufficient pulmonary arterial blood flow to lead to acute increases in pulmonary artery pressure with right ventricular strain, and to interrupt blood supply to distal segments of the lung.

Missed diagnoses are life-threatening because the mortality of untreated patients may be as high as 25–41%. PEs are often underdiagnosed in clinical practice, because they are frequently nonspecific in their clinical presentation. In one postmortem survey, PE was not suspected clinically in 70% of patients in whom it was subsequently shown to have been the major cause of death. However, overdiagnosis is also not without risk owing to the haemorrhagic hazards of the main treatment regime, anticoagulation; major bleeds occur in 1–10% of patients according to the degree of coexisting disease.

THE NATURAL HISTORY OF PEs

Once a thrombus has formed in the venous system, if it is not degraded by fibrinolysis or organized into the vascular wall, it may detach, migrate through the right heart to the pulmonary circulation, and impact in pulmonary arteries (**87**). A massive embolus, obstructing the main pulmonary arteries is usually fatal, but the majority of patients survive the initial PE. Studies from the preanticoagulation era suggested approximately 90% of patients survived a deep vein thrombosis (DVT), and three-quarters survived a PE. The initial thrombus may resolve spontaneously, by fibrinolysis. Rapid resolution of vascular obstruction may be observed after 6 days in man, and earlier in dogs, but often remains incomplete for weeks or months. Even if pulmonary arteries remain obliterated, the recruitment of alternative vascular channels can maintain the circulation.

The main risk for untreated patients is of further PEs, particularly if the source thrombus and risk factors are still present. A series of studies indicate recurrence rates of between 2–12%, and the risk of recurrence approaches 20% in patients presenting with hypotension and shock on the initial event. Any recurrence places the patient again at the risk of an acute massive and fatal PE. In addition, the patient is at risk of recurrent initial events that may obliterate sufficient numbers of pulmonary arteries to overwhelm the recruitment capacity, and lead to the development of chronic pulmonary hypertension and right heart failure.

RISK FACTORS FOR THE DEVELOPMENT OF PEs

PEs generally occur in settings of venous stasis, or other local or generalized alterations in the coagulation and fibrinolytic systems generating a prothrombotic state. Increasingly, genetic variations in these cascades are recognized as risk factors for thromboses (88a). These genetic variations (such as the Factor V Leiden mutation) are commonly found in the normal population, and individually each lead to only a small incremental risk.

It is when genetic risk factors are combined with acquired risk factors that PEs are most likely to develop; the exponential increase in PE incidence with age may reflect the development of more acquired risk factors. Well-substantiated clinical risk factors for DVTs and PEs are illustrated in figure **88b**. One or more of the first four classical predisposing factors shown in bold are present in 80–90% of patients. If no classical risk factors are apparent in a patient with a proven PE, then malignancy should be considered, and careful clinical assessment, chest radiography, and routine blood tests performed. More extensive investigations are only recommended if there are abnormalities on these initial tests.

CLINICAL FEATURES

Significant PEs are almost always accompanied by evidence of disturbed pulmonary vascular physiology:

- ❏ Evidence of elevated right atrial pressure (elevated jugular venous pressure [JVP]) in the majority of cases, and in massive or chronic thromboembolic disease, evidence of right ventricular strain (right ventricular [RV] heave, loud split P2, ECG or echocardiographic features).
- ❏ Arterial hypoxaemia or hypocapnic normoxaemia, due to deranged ventilation–perfusion (VQ) relationships as ventilated areas of the lung are no longer perfused.

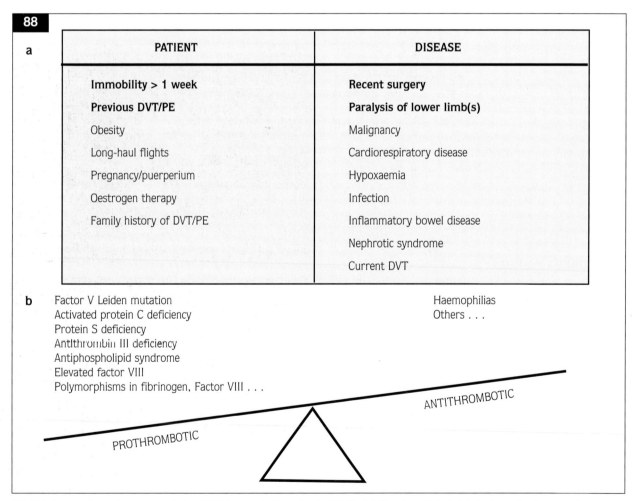

88

a

PATIENT	DISEASE
Immobility > 1 week	**Recent surgery**
Previous DVT/PE	**Paralysis of lower limb(s)**
Obesity	Malignancy
Long-haul flights	Cardiorespiratory disease
Pregnancy/puerperium	Hypoxaemia
Oestrogen therapy	Infection
Family history of DVT/PE	Inflammatory bowel disease
	Nephrotic syndrome
	Current DVT

b

Factor V Leiden mutation
Activated protein C deficiency
Protein S deficiency
Antithrombin III deficiency
Antiphospholipid syndrome
Elevated factor VIII
Polymorphisms in fibrinogen, Factor VIII . . .

Haemophilias
Others . . .

PROTHROMBOTIC

ANTITHROMBOTIC

88 Risk factors for pulmonary embolus (PE)/deep vein thrombosis (DVT). (**a**) Classical clinical risk factors; the four most common are in bold; (**b**) Genetic risk and protective factors

According to the size of the embolus, degree of pulmonary arterial bed obstruction, and underlying clinical state of the patient, three major clinical patterns are recognized:
❏ Collapse or shock +/- central chest pain.
❏ Pleuritic chest pain, haemoptysis, and dyspnoea.
❏ 'Isolated' dyspnoea.

Collapse or shock, with or without central chest pain

This scenario is seen in patients experiencing acute massive PEs (which account for approximately 5% of PEs). They generally impact in and occlude proximal pulmonary arteries (89), and include so-called 'saddle emboli', which obstruct both pulmonary arteries at the bifurcation of the pulmonary artery trunk. The degree of obstruction of the right ventricular outflow tract determines the severity of acute haemodynamic compromise. This may lead to cardiorespiratory arrest with pulse-less electrical activity – thromboembolus represents one of the 'four Ts' of the advanced life support (ALS) algorithm. In less severe cases, syncope or faintness may indicate a peri-arrest scenario.

In conscious patients dyspnoea is severe, and may be improved by lying flat (in contrast to other causes of acute dyspnoea). Patients may complain of central chest pain – any pleuritic pain is likely to relate to an earlier PE. Examination generally reveals cyanosis and tachypnoea in the absence of focal respiratory signs. Cardiac signs dominate the clinical picture: there will be evidence of a low cardiac output (elevated JVP, hypotension, tachycardia, and peripheral vasoconstriction) and often a right ventricular gallop rhythm. Oligaemic lung fields may be evident on chest radiograph (90). Cardiac investigations usually confirm the diagnosis with ECG evidence of right ventricular

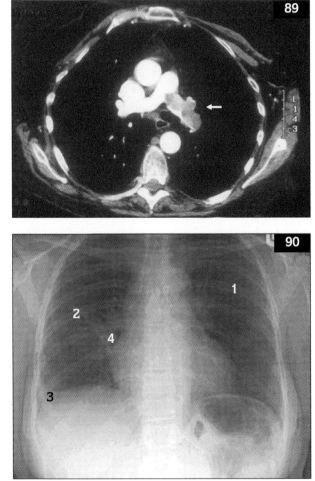

89 Massive pulmonary embolus. Near-occlusion of left main pulmonary arterial trunk by massive pulmonary embolus, demonstrated by helical CT scan with contrast. The embolus (arrowed) appears grey compared to the white contrast flowing through patent pulmonary arteries.

90 PA-chest radiograph of patient with bilateral massive pulmonary emboli. **1**. pulmonary oligaemia; **2**. plate atelectasis; **3**. pleural reaction; **4**. hilar prominence due to acutely dilated pulmonary arteries

strain (right bundle branch block [RBBB], T wave inversion in V1–4, and the frequently cited, but less commonly observed, full S1Q3T3 pattern (**91**)), and echocardiographic or CT demonstration of right ventricular dilatation and dysfunction.

Pleuritic chest pain, haemoptysis, and dyspnoea

This is the most common and best recognized pattern, accounting for approximately 60% of cases, and is caused by occlusion of segmental pulmonary arteries by small or medium-sized emboli. This results in infarction of areas of the lung parenchyma, inflammation of the overlying pleura, and often a low-grade fever. Examination often reveals a pleural rub, pleural effusion, and/or localized crackles. Any pleural effusion is usually blood-stained when aspirated, but aspiration should not be performed until a chest radiograph has confirmed that the clinical findings are due to an effusion rather than an elevated hemidiaphragm. The chest radiograph may also reveal segmental opacities or linear shadows (**90**), or may be apparently normal.

Pneumonia is the most important differential diagnosis, and is probably more common than PEs in this context, yet it is often overlooked as the initial diagnosis by students. Pneumonia should be considered more likely if the patient has a significant fever, purulent sputum, and raised white blood cells (WBC) and elevated C-reactive protein (CRP).

Isolated dyspnoea

In as many as a third of cases PEs lead to breathlessness without any other symptoms, usually as a result of showers of microemboli. Respiratory signs are minimal as pulmonary infarction is relatively rare (owing to the capacity of bronchial and pulmonary circulations to provide collateral supply through existing anastomotic channels), and there is initially little rise in pulmonary arterial pressure. In time, however, as increasing proportions of the pulmonary vascular bed are occluded, pulmonary arterial pressure rises, and signs of right ventricular strain and decompensation develop, representing thromboembolic pulmonary hypertension.

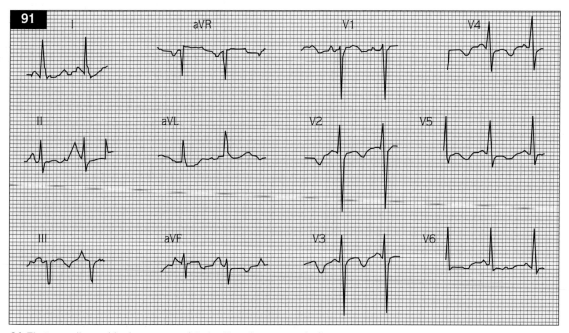

91 Electrocardiographic changes associated with pulmonary emboli

Individuals who already have chronically impaired cardiorespiratory reserve may decompensate with only relatively minor thromboembolic disease, in contrast to previously fit patients. Timely diagnosis of PEs in patients with pre-existing respiratory disease, such as COPD or pulmonary fibrosis, demands a high index of clinical suspicion and astute investigations.

INVESTIGATIONS AND DIAGNOSIS

While it is important that the diagnosis of PE is always considered, the clinical suspicion should not be high in patients without major risk factors, in whom alternative diagnoses are likely. PEs are confirmed in less than one third of clinically suspected cases. Crucial points in the examination and investigation of PE patients are summarized in *Table 63*. Since interpretation of certain tests is critically dependent upon the clinical likelihood of PE, there should be two steps to making a diagnosis:

❏ Determination of the degree of clinical suspicion based on whether a PE is likely, and whether alternative diagnoses are unlikely (**92**). All patients with a possible PE should have the pretest clinical probability recorded. *In the setting of a normal respiratory rate, jugular venous pressure, and PaO2, it is particularly important to consider alternative diagnoses.*

Table 63 Diagnosis of deep vein thrombosis (DVT) and pulmonary embolus (PE)

Clinical signs	Mandatory basic tests	Tests for DVTs	Specific tests for PE
Tachypnoeic	Chest radiograph	Doppler ultrasound	VQ scan
Cyanosed	ECG	venography	CT scan with contrast
Elevated JVP	Arterial blood gases		Echocardiography
Hypotensive	(D-dimers)		Pulmonary angiogram
Right ventricular heave			
Loud P2	FBC and CRP to exclude pneumonia		
Pleural rub	Baseline clotting screen		

CRP, C-reactive protein; CT, computed tomography; ECG, electrocardiogram; FBC, full blood count; JVP, jugular venous pressure; VQ, ventilation–perfusion

---

If PE is suspected   **92**

Are other diagnoses unlikely?

- Clinically and after basic tests
  - FBC
  - CXR
  - ECG
  - Spirometry/peak flow
  - Blood gases

YES   score + 1

Is a major risk factor present?

- Recent immobility
- Recent lower limb trauma/surgery
- Clinical DVT
- Previous proven DVT/PE
- Pregnancy or puerperium
- Major medical illness

YES   score + 1

	Score	2	1	0
	PE probability	High	Intermediate	Low
D-dimer test		No	Yes	Yes
(LMW) heparin		Yes	Yes	Wait
PE tests		Urgent	Early	Consider

92 Diagnostic algorithm for pulmonary embolus (PE); results which confirm or refute the diagnosis of PE are shown in bold boxes. If at any stage the results contradict the clinical impression, the advice of a senior colleague should be sought. CXR, chest X-ray; DVT, deep vein thrombosis; ECG, electrocardiogram; FBC, full blood count; LMW, low molecular weight

❏ Tests of diagnostic confirmation/exclusion (93) should be performed, according to the patients' condition. *Their use in particularly clinical settings is discussed after the next section which summarizes the individual diagnostic tests.*

The chest radiograph

The chest radiograph is often normal in PEs, a finding that may be important when considering other differential diagnoses for dyspnoeic patients. There are, however, abnormalities suggestive of PEs including segmental opacities, linear shadows, and pleural reactions (90). Bilateral horizontal linear shadows in the lower zones, with or without a pleural reaction, should prompt clinical suspicion of PEs whatever the context. More subtle changes include oligaemic lung fields, with areas of the lung hypertranslucent compared to the opposite side, and hilar prominence due to enlarged main pulmonary arteries.

Helical thoracic CT scan with contrast ('CT pulmonary angiography')

Helical thoracic CT scan using a PE protocol optimizes imaging of pulmonary arteries by acquiring images in a single breath hold, an appropriate time after the injection of intravenous contrast medium. To reduce radiation burden, apices and bases are not included. The 'spiral' of information is then reconstructed into contiguous axial sections. Such scans can demonstrate the presence of thrombus in proximal (89) and segmental pulmonary arteries. Subsegmental arterial thrombus is less readily seen, though good results are obtained from the latest scanners, with optimized protocols for contrast injection, and work-station scan reporting. If the pulmonary artery pressure has been elevated acutely, additional changes will be seen, including RV and right atrium (RA) dilatation, and reflux of contrast into the azygos vein. Mosaic perfusion may also be demonstrated. It is crucial to perform the scan as early as possible, and preferably within 24 hours as an abnormal scan may become normal within 1 week.

Ventilation–perfusion (VQ) scans

The cardinal feature of PEs on VQ scans are 'unmatched' perfusion defects, i.e. abnormalities of perfusion in areas of normal ventilation (94a). Ventilation is imaged by the distribution of an inhaled nonabsorbed radiolabelled gas: [81]krypton is preferable to [133]xenon. Pulmonary perfusion is imaged by studying the distribution of [99m]technetium-labelled albumin macroaggregates that impact in the pulmonary capillary

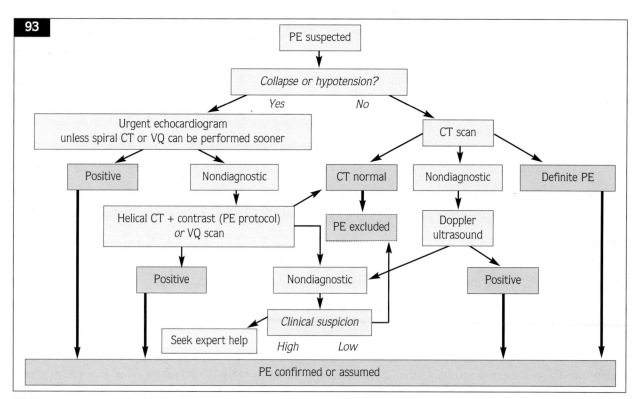

93 Clinical assessment of patient with suspected pulmonary embolus (PE). CT, computed tomography; VQ, ventilation–perfusion

94 Ventilation–perfusion (VQ) scan images in diagnosis of pulmonary emboli (PE). (**a**) VQ scan in patient with multiple PEs. Posterior views of lungs indicating ventilation (i) and perfusion (ii). Note multiple large defects of perfusion in areas of normal ventilation, with no perfusion to right lower zone, and 'moth eaten' appearance throughout left lung. (CT scan and CXR illustrated in **89** and **90**); (**b**) Modified PIOPED criteria for interpretation of VQ scans; (**c**) Clinical settings in which VQ scans will be difficult to interpret. COPD, chronic obstructive pulmonary disease; CXR, chest X-ray

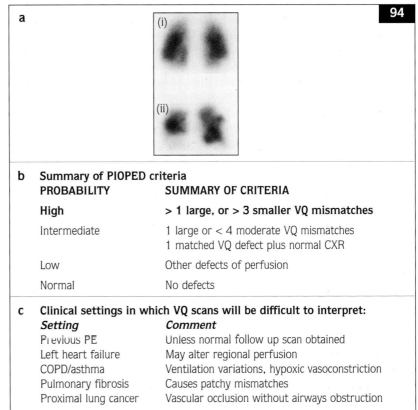

b   Summary of PIOPED criteria

PROBABILITY	SUMMARY OF CRITERIA
High	**> 1 large, or > 3 smaller VQ mismatches**
Intermediate	1 large or < 4 moderate VQ mismatches 1 matched VQ defect plus normal CXR
Low	Other defects of perfusion
Normal	No defects

c   Clinical settings in which VQ scans will be difficult to interpret:

Setting	*Comment*
Previous PE	Unless normal follow up scan obtained
Left heart failure	May alter regional perfusion
COPD/asthma	Ventilation variations, hypoxic vasoconstriction
Pulmonary fibrosis	Causes patchy mismatches
Proximal lung cancer	Vascular occlusion without airways obstruction

bed. The number and size of perfusion defects, in association with the chest radiographic appearance, are used to determine the probability that the scan appearances are due to pulmonary emboli (**94b**). The scan should be performed early as an abnormal VQ scan may become normal within 1 week. VQ scans carry good sensitivity and specificity to level of segmental and subsegmental arteries, but are difficult or impossible to interpret in certain patients (**94c**), in whom alternative diagnostic investigations should be used.

Evidence, particularly from the PIOPED study, indicates that a normal VQ scan reliably excludes PE, and is sufficient to refute or confirm the diagnosis of PE unless there is a disparate clinical opinion. A high probability scan in an appropriate setting offers good evidence that PE has occurred, but false positives may occur, particularly in patients with previous PEs. Unfortunately, most commonly the scan is nondiagnostic, reported as of low or intermediate probability for PEs. Up to a third of these patients may have PEs necessitating further investigation.

Echocardiography

An echocardiogram is essential if collapse is present or imminent. This may demonstrate the thrombus itself.

Cardiac signs suggestive of PE include right ventricular dilatation and hypokinesis, abnormal septal movement, and lack of inferior vena cava (IVC) collapse during inspiration. Importantly, echocardiography will exclude other cardiac conditions that may mimic acute massive PEs, such as aortic dissection, pericardial tamponade, or acute valvular or septal rupture.

Investigation of leg and pelvic veins

Of patients with an acute PE, 70% will have thrombus in proximal leg veins, often with no clinical evidence of DVT. Source thrombus in the proximal leg veins may be detected by serial compression ultrasonography with Doppler studies or contrast venography, reducing the need for lung imaging. A single negative study is insufficient, however, to exclude PE.

D-dimers

D-dimers are specific degradation products of cross-linked fibrin and are rarely found in the normal range of levels in patients with venous thromboembolism, since fibrinolytic cascades are activated. Elevated D-dimers cannot, however, be used as a confirmatory diagnostic test for PEs as they are increased in many clinical settings, including trauma, infection, and inflammation. Limitations with clinically available tests mean many clinicians remain cautious about D-dimers, but an entirely normal laboratory (not bedside) D-dimer test is a useful test to exclude PEs where the clinical suspicion of PEs is low; where there is moderate clinical suspicion of PEs, D-dimers should not be used alone to exclude PEs.

Formal pulmonary angiography

Formal pulmonary angiography is now rarely performed for the diagnosis of acute PE, as safer and quicker methods are available in the majority of centres. It continues to have a role for diagnosis of subsegmental thrombus and for interventional procedures.

DIAGNOSIS OF PES IN CLINICAL PRACTICE

The exact tests and diagnostic routes varies according to the patient's condition.

Investigation of acutely unwell patients with imminent collapse

The most useful investigation is usually an urgent echocardiogram, which may demonstrate the thrombus itself or cardiac signs suggestive of PE, and will exclude important differential cardiac diagnoses. If a helical CT scan or VQ scan can be obtained before an echocardiogram, then one of these should be performed urgently instead of echocardiography. According to local expertise and availability, formal pulmonary angiography may be appropriate, particularly if the patient has already followed a cardiac work-up with emergency coronary angiography.

Investigation of normotensive patients with suspected pulmonary embolism

More than 85% of cases will fall into this category. CT pulmonary angiograms (CTPA) using the latest generation of multislice scanners are now the recommended first line imaging investigation in the diagnosis of suspected pulmonary emboli, since they are readily available out of hours, quick to perform, carry good sensitivity and specificity to level of segmental arteries, and may be diagnostic for non PE. Until recently, VQ scans were the recommended first line investigation, and they remain a very useful tool in centres with appropriate expertise and standardized reporting criteria.

In practice, the main problems arise when there is a significant clinical suspicion of PEs, but the CT scan is reported as normal and the VQ scan is nondiagnostic. *In this situation, PEs have not been excluded* since subsegmental arterial thrombus is poorly detected by CTPA and VQ scans. Diagnosis of isolated subsegmental thrombus may be crucial, particularly in patients with pre-existing cardiorespiratory disease. The diagnosis may be inferred if source thrombus is detected in leg veins, and Doppler ultrasonography should be performed. If the CT scan, VQ scan, and Doppler studies are all negative but the clinical presentation is highly suggestive of PEs, experienced clinicians would still be reluctant to exclude PEs. Formal pulmonary angiography may be useful in this situation.

MANAGEMENT

The speed at which investigations are ordered and treatment commenced should be determined by the patient's condition and the degree of clinical suspicion that a PE is present. As noted in the British Thoracic Society (BTS)'s algorithm (92), formal treatment often needs to be instituted before the diagnosis of PE is confirmed.

General measures

Oxygen should be administered to hypoxaemic patients. The initial priority, particularly for hypotensive patients, is to restore and maintain the circulation. External cardiac massage in cardiopulmonary resuscitation may be particularly useful in patients with massive proximal PEs, in whom the occluding thrombus may be broken up and dissipated to multiple distal pulmonary arteries.

MASSIVE PES WITH CIRCULATORY COLLAPSE
Thrombolytic agents

Thrombolysis to disrupt and degrade existing thrombus is recommended for patients with massive PEs and circulatory collapse. A 50 mg bolus of altepase is recommended by the latest BTS guidelines, if cardiac arrest is imminent. If indicated, thrombolysis should be administered as soon as possible, and is unlikely to be effective if given after 14 days of the acute event when there is no residual lysis substrate (fresh plasminogen) in the clot.

The role of thrombolysis remains controversial in patients with lesser degrees of right ventricular dysfunction, for example dysfunction solely demonstrated by echocardiography. There is no indication to use thrombolysis in other clinical settings in which the haemorrhagic risks of thrombolysis outweigh the potential benefits.

Embolectomy

Surgical and catheter embolectomies in the setting of acute PE carry mortality rates too high for the

Table 64 Comparison of anticoagulation for pulmonary embolus using heparins and warfarin

	Heparins	Warfarin
Route of administration	IV/SC	Oral
Time for anticoagulation	Immediate	3 days
Usually measure efficacy by	APTT (UFH); nil (LMWH)	INR
Usual duration	~5 days	≥ 3 months
Reversal	Protamine (UFH); LMWH. Discuss with your haematologist	Vitamin K; factor concentrates

APTT, activated partial thromboplastin time; INR, internation normalized ratio; LMWH, low molecular weight heparin; UFH, unfractionated heparin

Table 65 Benefits and relative contraindications to the use of low molecular weight heparins

Advantages of low molecular weight heparins in treatment of pulmonary embolus (PE)

❏ Predictable dose response

❏ Blood monitoring not routinely indicated

❏ Subcutaneous administration – no need for intravenous infusions

❏ Superior side-effect profile to unfractionated heparin

❏ At least equivalent efficacy for PE treatment

Situations in which intravenous unfractionated heparin may be preferable

❏ If reversal of anticoagulation is likely to be needed rapidly (e.g. surgery, unstable patient)

❏ For obese patients (weight–dose correlations do not hold)

❏ In renal impairment if estimated creatinine clearance is < 50 ml/minute

procedures to be to considered in any but moribund patients in whom the diagnosis of PE is absolutely confirmed. Fragmenting a massive embolus in the main pulmonary arteries using a pigtail catheter may be used in preference.

NONMASSIVE PES
Anticoagulation

Anticoagulation is used to prevent extension and recurrence of the thrombus. Baseline clotting studies (activated partial thromboplastics time [APTT] and prothrombin time [PTR]) and bloods for thrombophilia screens should be taken before anticoagulation is commenced. Rapid anticoagulation is achieved using heparin, levels of which need to be therapeutic within 24 hours for full efficacy. Heparin also provides an easily reversible means of anticoagulation in patients in whom PEs are suspected but not yet proven. Long-term anticoagulation in patients with proven PEs is usually

achieved using oral warfarin to antagonize vitamin K; however, for patients with a proven PE, heparin should be continued until warfarin has resulted in a stable international normalized ratio (INR) within the therapeutic range. *Table 64* indicates the major differences between heparin and warfarin.

Following a single PE, patients should receive at least a 3 month course, particularly if there was no known, temporary precipitating risk factor. The length of anticoagulation courses for patients with a single event but ongoing risk factors will vary according to clinical circumstances. Warfarin can be discontinued only if there is no clinical evidence of recurrence or pulmonary hypertension at the end of the intended course. Two PEs demand life-long anticoagulation, unless the risks of anticoagulation are deemed excessive in a particular patient.

Heparins

Heparin should be started immediately for patients with an intermediate or high clinical suspicion of PE. Two forms of heparin are in clinical use – unfractionated heparin and the more recently developed low molecular weight (LMW) heparins such as tinzaparin, enoxaparin, and dalteparin.

Low molecular weight (LMW) heparin: The past few years have seen a switch from intravenous unfractionated heparin to subcutaneous low molecular weight heparin. This was primarily driven by the difficulties in establishing therapeutic heparinization at 24 hours. Accumulating evidence indicates that LMW heparins are as effective as unfractionated heparin, and there are many additional clinical reasons for their preference to IV heparin (*Table 65*). Doses of LMW heparins are calculated on the basis of patient weight; for example the treatment dose of enoxaparin is 100 units/kg, and for tinzaparin 175 units/kg. Therapeutic efficacy is not routinely measured, but if assays are required (for example in pregnancy or renal impairment), the anti-Xa to anti-IIa ratio can be used.

Unfractionated heparin: There are, however, situations in which an intravenous infusion of unfractionated heparin should still be used in preference to LMW heparins (*Table 65*, page 143). It is a useful first dose bolus and the action of heparin can readily be reversed and restarted. The half-life of < 2 hours means that stopping the infusion is usually sufficient to reverse anticoagulation; protamine should only be used under expert guidance from the haematology services. It is crucially important to obtain early therapeutic levels and to avoid over-anticoagulation, placing the patient at a severe risk of haemorrhage. After 4–6 hours' treatment the APTT must be checked: if it is therapeutic, daily checks are required but any dose adjustments necessitate further APTT checks 4–6 hours later. If heparins are prescribed for more than 5 days, regular FBCs to check for heparin-induced thrombocytopenia are mandatory.

Warfarin
Warfarin should be started as soon as there is a confirmed diagnosis of PE. The INR should be checked each day after starting treatment until stable control is obtained, when weekly and eventually monthly checks will suffice, unless clinical circumstances change. The usual dosing schedule will start at 10 mg, before adjusting to a regular daily dose which will usually be between 3 and 10 mg. The initial dose should be lower (5 mg or less) in patients with elevated INR, liver disease, elderly patients, or patients with cardiac failure. Warfarin is teratogenic and should not be given during pregnancy. LMWH should be administered in preference, with the switch occurring before 6 weeks gestation.

All patients receiving warfarin need to be given careful advice to optimize their safety. They should be warned to carry the Department of Health anticoagulant booklet at all times, and to advise all doctors or pharmacists suggesting new treatments to check for warfarin interactions. They should also be told to seek urgent medical advice if they have reason to suspect over-anticoagulation (suggested by bleeding or bruising), or under-treatment, if tablets are missed, or diarrhoea or vomiting has occurred. Since drug interactions can lead to severe derangements that are not always predictable, a wise suggestion is to obtain an INR check a few days after the institution of any new treatment.

Other measures
Inferior vena cava filters should be considered for patients in whom recurrent PEs occur in spite of adequate anticoagulation. Filters are placed in the inferior vena cava, via jugular or femoral vein cannulation. The true long-term complication and success rates of such devices have not been fully determined, and all patients should receive careful follow-up.

FOLLOW-UP OF PATIENTS WITH PULMONARY EMBOLI
In addition to having careful follow-up in an anticoagulation clinic, PE patients need medical follow-up to ensure that pulmonary hypertension resolves. If clinical signs persist, further VQ scans can be helpful in distinguishing between residual or new disease. In either case, anticoagulation should be continued. If further PEs have occurred in spite of adequate anticoagulation, consideration of inferior vena cava filter devices is warranted.

Following an abnormal VQ scan, it is helpful to see evidence of the scan returning to normal, as this allows VQ scans to be more useful in the diagnostic work-up of any future suspected PEs.

PREVENTION OF DVT AND PE
Prophylaxis should be considered for all patients in whom venous stasis and hypercoagulable states are likely, including any patient hospitalized for more than 24–48 hours. Attention has tended to focus on surgical inpatients, but recent data indicate that in medical inpatients, DVT incidences of approximately 15–20% can be reduced by half by appropriate prophylaxis.

First-line prophylaxis consists of early ambulation, lower limb exercises for bed-bound patients, and prescription of graduated compression elastic stockings. The latter come in different sizes and should be fitted to avoid a tourniquet effect at the top of the stocking. Subcutaneous administration of low-dose heparin should be started before the risk of thrombosis develops, and continued for 6–10 days. Once-daily administration of LMW heparins is commonly used for convenience (e.g. enoxaparin 2,000–4,000 units, tinzaparin 3,500–4,500 units).

PULMONARY OEDEMA
Pulmonary oedema most commonly occurs following a large anterior myocardial infarction (MI) leading to left heart failure: acute elevations in left atrial pressure lead to acute pulmonary venous hypertension, precipitating pulmonary oedema. A

wide variety of additional pathologies lead to pulmonary oedema. Although the phrase 'noncardiogenic pulmonary oedema' is often used, it does not refer to all of the noncardiac causes and should be used with caution.

Pulmonary oedema develops if normal lymphatic clearance mechanisms that clear fluid from the interstitium are overwhelmed (95). Fluid flux from capillaries to the interstitial spaces is based on considerations given by Starling's principle:

$$\text{Fluid flux} = \frac{\text{filtration}}{\text{coefficient}} \times [\{\text{hydrostatic gradient}\} - \{\text{osmotic gradient}\}]$$

The aetiological mechanisms operating in pulmonary oedema are usefully divided into whether pressure changes or altered vascular wall permeability due to endothelial cell injury are primarily responsible for the oedema (*Table 66*). Hydrostatic pulmonary oedema can resolve extremely quickly if the underlying cause can be treated. Long-term consequences are rare,

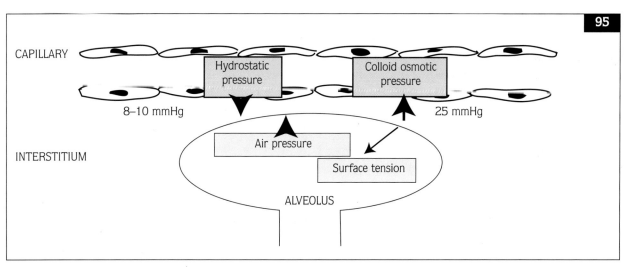

95 Pulmonary oedema. Diagram to show factors governing formation of oedema fluid when the pulmonary capillary bed is intact. Excess interstitial fluid drains to lymph channels

Table 66 Common causes of pulmonary oedema

Relative increase in hydrostatic pressure	Capillary leak syndrome
❏ Increased hydrostatic pressure	❏ Septicaemia
Acute myocardial infarction	❏ Aspiration
– usually large anterior MI	❏ Trauma and burns
– if inferior or posterior MI, consider acute MR	❏ Drugs
Mitral stenosis	Aspirin/opiate overdose
– and other forms of left atrial obstruction	Streptokinase
Volume overload with poor renal function	Hydrochlorthiazide
❏ Reduced colloid osmotic pressure	IV beta agonists
Hypoalbuminaemia	❏ Fat embolism
	❏ Lung ischaemia/reperfusion
	❏ Lung re-expansion

MI, myocardial infarction; MR, mitral regurgitation

unless the pulmonary capillary pressure rises sufficiently (> 30 mmHg) to force red blood cells into the interstitium resulting in pulmonary haemosiderosis. If pulmonary oedema results from capillary leakage, however, proteins and cellular debris will be present in the oedema fluid. This leads to coagulation of the oedema fluid and development of hyaline membranes, with important consequences for immediate management and long-term pulmonary damage.

CLINICAL FEATURES

Acute pulmonary oedema

Severe breathlessness in a grey, clammy patient coughing frothy sputum is the classical presentation of pulmonary oedema due to acute left ventricular failure. Inspiratory crackles will be evident at least in lower and mid zones. The patient will be hypoxaemic.

The precise clinical features will vary according to the underlying cause. For example, in the setting of both acute MI and septic shock, there will be hypotension and tachycardia. However, the patient with acute left ventricular failure will usually be grey and peripherally vasoconstricted, whereas the patient with septic shock will be peripherally vasodilated and may have bounding pulses. Usually the JVP is elevated in 'cardiac' causes, though, as this reflects right, not left, atrial pressure, there is no direct correlation between JVP and pulmonary oedema.

Mild or chronic pulmonary oedema

Patients with lesser degrees of pulmonary oedema complain of breathlessness on exertion, orthopnoea, and paroxysmal nocturnal dyspnoea. Inspiratory crackles will be audible at the bases of the lungs. There are usually no gross haemodynamic changes.

Investigations and diagnosis

Initial investigations should include CXR, ECG, FBC, urine and electrolytes, and cardiac enzymes. In a breathless patient in whom pulmonary oedema is suspected, a chest radiograph series will be diagnostic. If there is a very rapid improvement in the appearance of the chest radiographs (i.e. within minutes or hours), the diagnosis is likely to be pulmonary oedema.

The chest radiograph abnormalities associated with pulmonary oedema can be understood from physiological principles:

Cardiogenic pulmonary oedema

The chest radiograph changes reflect progressive increases in pulmonary venous pressure. Mild elevation (between 15 and 20 mmHg) results in vascular dilatation and is seen on the chest radiograph as dilated upper lobe pulmonary veins and dilated main pulmonary arteries. As the pulmonary venous pressure rises further, interstitial oedema develops, leading to thickened interlobular septa and dilated lymphatics; these appear as horizontal lines in the costophrenic angles, and are known as 'septal' or 'Kerley B' lines. Even higher pulmonary venous pressures, exceeding 30 mmHg, result in alveolar oedema. The chest radiograph then displays 'diffuse bilateral alveolar infiltrates' (hazy opacification spreading out from the hila), and pleural effusions. With cardiogenic pulmonary oedema, the cardio-thoracic ratio is likely to be increased.

Other causes of pulmonary oedema

In pulmonary oedema of other causes, the early changes are often not observed, and the chest radiograph changes usually reflect the interstitial or alveolar oedema changes.

MANAGEMENT

Patients with acute pulmonary oedema should be treated in a high-dependency unit, initially in the accident and emergency unit, and thereafter on a coronary care or other designated high-dependency unit. Appropriate management is crucially dependent on identifying the cause of the pulmonary oedema. Most commonly, acute pulmonary oedema will be due to an acute MI and the diagnosis will be obvious from clinical history and ECG. Noncardiac management has important differences (see below).

Acute pulmonary oedema due to left ventricular failure

A patient with acute pulmonary oedema associated with left heart failure will be terrified if still conscious, and will need emergency treatment. They should be sat up to reduce pulmonary congestion, given high-flow, high-concentration oxygen via a face mask, and given intravenous morphine. While the latter is a painkiller and may help any co-existing cardiac pain, in this setting it is used to alleviate breathlessness and reverse reflex vasoconstriction. An intravenous loop diuretic – such as furosemide 40–80 mg – may provide rapid relief via its vasodilator properties.

If these immediate measures fail, a senior colleague needs to be contacted, as inotropic support, further vasodilators, and ventilation may be required. Positive pressure ventilation, usually via CPAP, permits the use of positive end expiratory pressure to drive oedema fluid back into the circulation. Measurement of central venous pressure may be helpful, particularly if the cause is in doubt, though there have been moves away from diagnostic pulmonary artery catheterization.

Noncardiac pulmonary oedema
Senior help is urgently required as prompt treatment of the precipitating cause is crucial in the management of this condition, and the underlying cause may not be evident. Most patients will fulfil the oxygenation criteria for acute respiratory distress syndrome (ARDS) and require admission to intensive care for supplementary oxygen, mechanical ventilation (noninvasive and invasive), and judicious fluid and haematological management. Management is directed towards maintaining adequate oxygenation while minimizing further damage to the lung parenchyma by barotrauma (precipitated by the high ventilatory pressures that are usually required), infection, or haemodynamic disturbances.

PULMONARY HYPERTENSION
DEFINITION
Pulmonary hypertension (PH) is defined as a mean pulmonary artery pressure exceeding 25 mmHg. Elevated pulmonary arterial pressures are sustained at the expense of progressive hypertrophy of the RV and proximal pulmonary arteries, and ultimately right ventricular dilatation and failure (96). In the UK, in a patient with no obvious cardiac or respiratory pathology, the most common causes of moderate to severe PH will be thromboembolic PH due to chronic PEs, and primary PH.

Patients present with progressive breathlessness out of proportion to the severity of any precipitating underlying respiratory or cardiac disease, but the diagnosis is often elusive. If untreated the process is progressive, but improvements can occur if an underlying cause can be identified and corrected, or appropriate medical management instituted for responsive patients. Unfortunately, the diagnosis is often missed for many years.

AETIOLOGY
PH develops when the normal compensatory mechanisms that operate to keep pulmonary arterial pressures low are overwhelmed, and pulmonary vascular resistance cannot be sufficiently lowered by recruitment of previously underperfused capillaries.

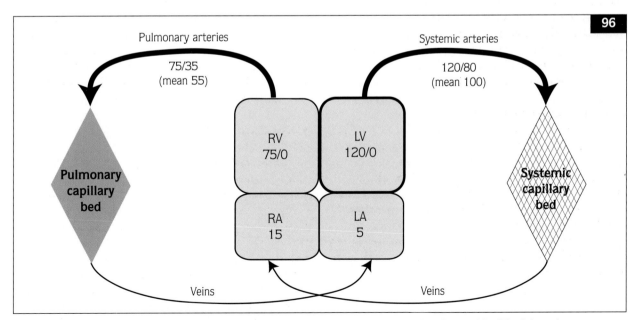

96 Diagram to show circulation in pulmonary hypertension (mmHg). LA, left atrium; LV, left ventricle; RA, right atrium; RV, right ventricle

Historically, PH has been divided into primary pulmonary hypertension (PPH) and secondary aetiologies. Secondary PH is usually due to cardiac or respiratory disease. Rarer causes are listed in *Table 67*, the latest classification according to the World Health Organization, which highlights the disparate pathologies that lead to PH. Mechanisms by which PH develops can be categorized as:

❑ Destruction of the pulmonary vascular bed:
  – Obliteration of vascular lumen (thrombo-embolus, intimal thickening [PPH]).
  – Loss of parenchymal lung tissue (e.g. emphysema).
❑ Chronic pressure or volume overload of the pulmonary circulation:
  – Pressure overload (e.g. left-to-right shunts of congenital heart disease).
  – Volume overload: sustained elevations of cardiac output (e.g. liver disease).
❑ Sustained elevations in pulmonary venous pressure, most commonly due to elevated left atrial pressure (e.g. left ventricular failure, mitral stenosis).
❑ Sustained hypoxic vasoconstriction in the absence of 'normal' areas of the vascular bed to which to divert flow (e.g. atmospheric hypoxia, generalized lung disease, such as fibrosis, emphysema).

CARDIAC CAUSES OF PH
Ischaemic and valvular heart disease are common cardiac conditions in the adult which can lead to PH. Left-sided atrial or ventricular heart disease of whatever cause (usually secondary to ischaemic heart disease) leads to elevated left atrial pressures, resulting in elevated pulmonary venous pressures. Thus 'biventricular failure' can result from purely left-sided cardiac pathology. Pulmonary venous pressure is also elevated by left-sided valvular heart disease, such as mitral stenosis.

Congenital heart disease can also lead to PH, though different mechanisms operate in such patients as a result of left-to-right shunts. An abnormal flow of intracardiac blood from left to right ventricles in a ventricular septal defect (VSD), or from aorta to pulmonary artery through a patent ductus arteriosus (PDA) results in high pulmonary artery pressures. In a subgroup of these patients, progressive obliteration of distal pulmonary vessels and other vascular remodelling events lead to further elevation of pulmonary artery pressures. Subsequent correction of the VSD or PDA usually fails to normalize pulmonary artery pressures. Eisenmenger's syndrome (reversal of the original left-to-right shunt) may develop and is characterized by more profound central cyanosis, and the development of digital clubbing.

In patients with sustained pulmonary artery volume overload from atrial septal defects (ASD), pulmonary arterial pressure is initially normal, but rises following remodelling of the pulmonary vascular bed in a subgroup of patients. Again, PH often persists following surgical correction of the initial defect, and Eisenmenger's syndrome may develop.

COR PULMONALE
Cor pulmonale is defined as right ventricular hypertrophy resulting from chronic lung disease, and is effectively due to the development of PH. Several pathogenic mechanisms are likely to contribute to the aetiology of PH in chronic lung diseases such as COPD, including sustained alveolar hypoxia, compression of capillaries in hyperinflated lungs, and intravascular flow impairment due to polycythaemia or thromboemboli. In emphysema there may also be direct destruction of the pulmonary vascular bed.

The development of peripheral oedema in a patient with COPD is dreaded by the informed patient, and for good reason, as it signifies that their pulmonary disease has probably progressed to a stage when PH has developed. However, in addition to patients with inexorably progressive disease, patients with chronic lung disease often develop intermittent RV failure. In a previously stable patient without clinical evidence of cor pulmonale, the development of peripheral oedema and other evidence of right heart failure should lead to the suspicion of an acute (and usually reversible) precipitant of PH:

❑ Intercurrent infection – particularly in patients with COPD. Alveolar hypoxia in nonventilated airways needs prompt treatment with physiotherapy.
❑ Pulmonary emboli: classical signs may be minimal as only small emboli are needed.
❑ New onset atrial fibrillation.
❑ Deteriorating left ventricular function following a silent MI.

THROMBOEMBOLIC PH
Chronic pulmonary emboli lead to progressive PH as described in the sections above. Similarly, nonresolved acute pulmonary emboli result in sustained elevation of pulmonary artery pressures. These are important diagnoses to make as therapies differ substantially (particularly from that of PPH, with which the chronic presentation can be confused).

Table 67 Classification of pulmonary hypertension according to the World Health Organization, 1998

1 Pulmonary arterial hypertension
- ❏ Primary pulmonary hypertension
  - Sporadic
  - Familial
- ❏ Pulmonary arterial hypertension related to:
  - Collagen vascular disease
  - Congenital systemic to pulmonary shunts
  - Portal hypertension
  - HIV infection
  - Drugs/toxins:
    - – anorexigens (aminorex, fenfluramine, dexfenfluramine)
    - – other, including toxic rapeseed oil
  - Persistent pulmonary hypertension of the newborn

2 Pulmonary venous hypertension
- ❏ Left-sided atrial or ventricular heart disease
- ❏ Left-sided valvular heart disease
- ❏ Pulmonary veno-occlusive disease
- ❏ Pulmonary capillary haemangiomatosis
- ❏ Other

3 Pulmonary hypertension associated with respiratory disorders and/or hypoxaemia
- ❏ Chronic obstructive lung disease
- ❏ Interstitial lung disease
- ❏ Sleep disordered breathing
- ❏ Alveolar hypoventilation disorders
- ❏ Chronic exposure to high altitude
- ❏ Neonatal lung disease
- ❏ Alveolar capillary dysplasia

4 Pulmonary hypertension due to chronic thrombotic and/or embolic disease
- ❏ Thrombo-embolic obstruction of proximal pulmonary arteries
- ❏ Obstruction of distal pulmonary arteries:
  - Pulmonary embolism (thrombus, tumour and so on)
  - *In situ* thrombosis
  - Sickle cell disease

5 Pulmonary hypertension associated with miscellaneous diseases
- ❏ Inflammatory (including schistosomiasis, sarcoidosis)
- ❏ Extrinsic compression of the central pulmonary veins:
  - Fibrosing mediastinitis
  - Lymphadenopathy/tumours

PRIMARY PULMONARY HYPERTENSION

PPH affects 1–2 per 1,000,000 individuals and is twice as common in women as in men. Endothelial and smooth muscle cell proliferation in pulmonary arterioles leads to thickening of the walls and the formation of plexiform lesions that occlude the vascular lumen. *In situ* thromboses contribute to the occlusion. Ultimately these changes lead to an increased pulmonary vascular resistance, right ventricular hypertrophy, dilatation, and failure. If untreated, the median survival is less than 3 years. Heart–lung transplantation is the only cure, but in recent years administration of vasodilators, particularly prostacyclin analogues, has been shown to greatly improve survival.

PPH remains a diagnosis of exclusion, though this may alter with the recent delineation of the molecular basis of familial PPH (which is due to germ-line mutations in the *BMPR2* gene). PPH may be precipitated by exposure of susceptible individuals to specific toxins, such as appetite suppressant drugs and rapeseed oil. Pathological processes highly similar to those in PPH occur in patients with collagen vascular diseases, HIV infection, and portal hypertension. Many individuals 'susceptible' to the development of PPH in these clinical settings will have mutations in *BMPR2*, but the degree to which these agents should be viewed as triggers of PPH rather than causative agents in their own right remains a subject of research.

CLINICAL FEATURES

Patients with pulmonary hypertension present with progressive breathlessness out of proportion to the severity of any precipitating underlying respiratory or cardiac disease.

Haemoptysis occurs as a result of the increased pulmonary capillary pressure. Patients may have anginal chest pains due to ischaemia of the hypertrophied RV. Examination should suggest the presence of PH: cyanosis, a resting tachycardia, elevated JVP with prominent a and v waves, RV heave, and a loud pulmonary second sound – masked if triscuspid regurgitation develops – all suggest the presence of significant PH. Peripheral oedema and ascites may be present. Additional signs will reflect the nature of any precipitating disease.

INVESTIGATIONS AND DIAGNOSIS

Routine tests performed in breathless patients which should suggest the possibility of PH include:

❑ Chest radiograph: the first radiographic sign of significant PH is usually enlarged main pulmonary arteries (the right lower pulmonary artery should be < 16 mm wide [97]). 'Pruning' of peripheral vascular markings may be evident. Although right ventricular hypertrophy and dilatation may be present, this may not be apparent from the radiographic cardiac silhouette until late in the disease.

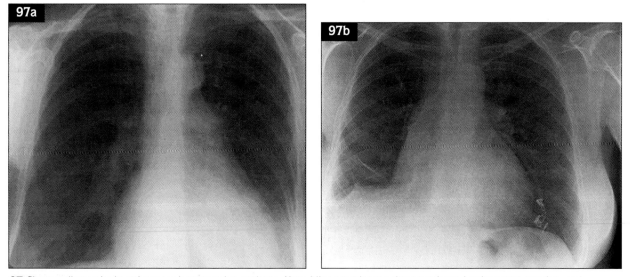

97 Chest radiographs in pulmonary hypertension patients. Note hilar prominence due to enlarged pulmonary arteries, and enlarged cardiac silhouette in **b**. Patient **b** also has pulmonary arteriovenous malformations which have been treated by right lower lobectomy and embolization: embolization coils are evident in the left lower zone

❏ ECG: features of right atrial and ventricular hypertrophy will be evident including RBBB, P pulmonale, T wave inversion in V1–4, and the full S1Q3T3 pattern (**91**).

❏ Arterial oxygen saturation and blood gases: severe hypoxaemia (SaO_2 < 90%, PaO_2 < 8 kPa) will usually be evident, accompanied by low normal $PaCO_2$.

❏ Thoracic CT scan: The most obvious abnormality occurs if the cross sections of the aorta and main pulmonary artery trunk are compared: the diameter of the pulmonary artery should be significantly less than that of the aorta, but in PH the pulmonary artery trunk diameter may equal or exceed the aortic diameter (**98**). A relative paucity of peripheral vascular markings may be evident. The hypertrophied or dilated right-sided chambers, with associated septal abnormalities, should be evident, and a pericardial effusion may be present.

❏ Lung function: in the absence of additional respiratory disease, spirometry (FEV_1, VC, and FEV_1/VC ratio) and lung volumes (TLC, RV) should be normal, except in late stages of the disease. The crucial abnormality is seen on assessment of gas transfer: the TLCO and KCO will be severely reduced (< 70% predicted), reflecting the reduced microvascular bed available for gas exchange.

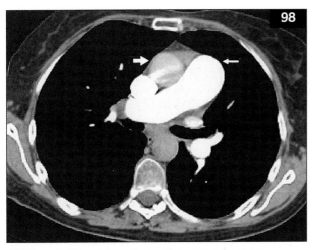

98 Thoracic CT scan in patient with severe pulmonary hypertension. Note that the contrast-filled pulmonary artery trunk (small arrow) has a diameter exceeding that of the aorta (large arrow) at the same level

SPECIALIZED TESTS TO DIAGNOSE AND QUANTIFY PH
Echocardiography

Wall thickness and overall dimensions of the right-sided cardiac chambers on two-dimensional echocardiography will suggest the presence of PH. A simple test to support the diagnosis can be performed by Doppler analysis of the tricuspid regurgitant jet of blood (detectable even if not evident on clinical examination). The maximum flow velocity of the jet depends on the pressure gradient across the valve: as the right atrial pressure can be estimated from the JVP, the right ventricular pressure and hence pulmonary artery pressure can be estimated. Additional specialized tests are also performed.

Cardiac catheterization

Direct pressure measurements are made using a pulmonary artery catheter; pulmonary arterial and right-sided cardiac chamber pressures are measured directly by appropriate catheter tip placement. Pulmonary venous pressure is measured during brief balloon occlusions of the pulmonary arterial flow. Catheterization allows a calculation of the cardiac output (using Fick's haemodilution method) and the pulmonary vascular resistance, which is important in determining the prognosis. Finally, catheterization allows a therapeutic test of the response of the pulmonary circulation to acute administration of vasodilator substances (see below).

MANAGEMENT

Any reversible cause or factor exacerbating PH should be treated. Patients should avoid strenuous exercise, pregnancy, and high altitude, which can further increase pulmonary arterial pressure. Administration of long-term oxygen in severely hypoxaemic patients and anticoagulation each prolong survival. In patients with severe PH due to chronic thromboembolic disease with proximal obstruction, surgical thromboendarterectomy may be possible, and carries a lower mortality than heart–lung transplantation, the only 'cure'.

In recent years administration of vasodilators, particularly prostacyclin analogues, has been shown to improve survival greatly in PPH. The effect of prostacyclin therapy on exercise tolerance varies from inhibition of deterioration to up to a 30% improvement on the pre-treatment baseline. The approval of the endothelin antagonist, bosentan, for PPH offers another option for improving haemodynamics and vascular remodelling in this condition.

PULMONARY ARTERIOVENOUS MALFORMATIONS AND RIGHT-TO-LEFT SHUNTS

Physiological shunts are essential for the maintenance of ventilation and perfusion relationships; if alveoli are not aerated owing to airway obstruction, oedema fluid or other pathology, then physiological hypoxic vasoconstriction diverts pulmonary blood flow to other aerated areas (**99a**). In pathological right-to-left shunts, pulmonary arterial blood is not diverted to other areas of the lung, but instead returns direct to the left atrium (**99b**).

Pathological right-to-left shunts occur most commonly in pulmonary arteriovenous malformations (PAVMs). Intrapulmonary right-to-left shunts are also seen in the hepatopulmonary syndrome in patients with severe liver disease. In Eisenmenger's syndrome, due to reversal of left-to-right shunts of congenital heart disease, the right-to-left shunts are nonpulmonary (**99b**).

Capillary-free communications between the pulmonary and systemic circulations have two important clinical consequences:

❏ Pulmonary arterial blood passing through these right-to-left shunts cannot be oxygenated, leading to hypoxaemia.

❏ The absence of a filtering capillary bed allows particulate matter to reach the systemic circulation, where it impacts in other capillary beds causing clinical sequelae, particularly in the cerebral circulation.

Massive right-to-left shunts may be recognized by the clinical triad of profound central cyanosis, digital clubbing, and polycythaemia.

PULMONARY ARTERIOVENOUS MALFORMATIONS

PAVMs are abnormal intrapulmonary vascular structures that develop postnatally (usually in puberty). PAVMs occur sporadically, but over 90% of PAVMs occur in association with the inherited disorder hereditary haemorrhagic telangiectasia (HHT, or Osler–Weber–Rendu syndrome). The discussion below focuses on these noniatrogenic PAVMs, in which historical mortality rates ranged from 4 to 40%. PAVMs also occur in patients in whom cyanotic congenital heart disease has been corrected by surgically-generated cavopulmonary or atriopulmonary shunts.

CLINICAL FEATURES

Approximately 50% of patients have no respiratory symptoms at the time of presentation, even with physical signs, such as cyanosis, clubbing, a vascular bruit, or abnormal chest radiographs. The commonest symptom is dyspnoea, but this may not be appreciated until after the condition has been treated. PAVM patients even tolerate worsening hypoxaemia on exercise well, reflecting their low pulmonary vascular resistance and ability to generate a supranormal cardiac output, which may increase further on exercise. Pleuritic chest pain of uncertain aetiology occurs in up to 10% of patients. A similar percentage experience haemoptysis, which may be due to accompanying endobronchial telangiectasia. The majority of patients with PAVMs will have personal or family evidence of underlying HHT, though this may require careful questioning.

Patients with clinically silent right-to-left shunts are still at risk of major complications. Haemorrhage from the PAVMs may be fatal during pregnancy, and catastrophic embolic cerebral events (cerebral abscess and embolic stroke) and transient ischaemic attacks occur in patients regardless of the degree of respiratory symptoms.

INVESTIGATIONS AND DIAGNOSIS

Most PAVM patients are hypoxaemic, reflecting their right-to-left shunt, but the differential diagnosis of

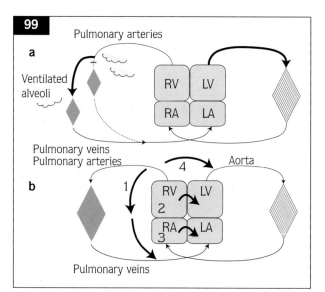

99 Shunts. (a) Physiological intrapulmonary shunting due to hypoxic vasoconstriction (dotted line bars) directs pulmonary arterial flow to aerated regions of the lung, and does not result in a right-to-left shunt; **(b)** Right-to-left shunts due to intrapulmonary (1) or intracardiac (reversed VSD [2] or ASD [3]) communications, or a reversed patent ductus arteriosus (4). ASD, atrial septal defect; LA, left atrium; LV, left ventricle; RA, right atrium; RV, right ventricle; VSD, ventricular septal defect

hypoxaemia is wide, and the degree of hypoxaemia may be subtle, even in the presence of clinically significant PAVMs. Formal diagnostic methods are based on noninvasive techniques to image the PAVMs and/or detect the right-to-left shunt.

Thoracic imaging

Chest radiographic appearance ranges from apparent normality, particularly if PAVMs are small or in the lower lobes where they can be obscured by a hemidiaphragm, through prominent bronchovascular markings, to the classical rounded mass with visible feeding or draining vessels. Helical CT scans detect smaller lesions (**100a**) and usefully exclude other diagnoses in hypoxaemic patients.

Right-to-left shunt quantification

Flow through anatomical intrapulmonary shunts can be detected and quantified by impaired oxygenation following inhalation of 100% oxygen for 20 minutes, or by a standard perfusion scan. The latter assesses the distribution of ^{99}mtechnetium-labelled albumin macroaggregates which should impact in the pulmonary capillary bed, but can pass through shunt vessels (**100b**). Quantifying the activity from the kidneys compared to the total dose injected provides the means for accurate quantification of the shunt. Contrast echocardiography can be used to detect the shunt, and allows exclusion of intracardiac shunting.

MANAGEMENT

PAVM complications can be limited if the condition is recognized and treated, with transcatheter embolization therapy offering the safest method of treatment. In experienced centres there are proven long-term physiological benefits of embolization, with excellent safety profiles, and this has supported the trend towards earlier treatment of the asymptomatic patient, accompanied by clinical screening of high-risk groups. In addition, prophylactic antibiotics are recommended at the time of dental and surgical procedures to reduce the risk of brain abscess. However, many PAVM patients remain undiagnosed, or under regular follow-up in respiratory units without consideration of intervention.

THE IMPORTANCE OF RECOGNIZING UNDERLYING HHT

Diagnosis and treatment of any PAVM is only one part of the management of a PAVM patient, more than 90% of whom will have underlying HHT, and it is crucial for the patient and their family that the physician is alert to this possibility. HHT is more commonly recognized by the consequences of abnormal dilated vessels developing in the systemic circulation, leading to epistaxes, mucocutaneous telangiectasia, and iron deficiency anaemia secondary to chronic gastrointestinal and/or nasal haemorrhage. Large arteriovenous malformations also occur in several systemic vascular beds, such as the cerebral, spinal, and hepatic circulations. Current clinical criteria for a definitive diagnosis of HHT require the presence of three out of four key features, namely: (1) spontaneous recurrent epistaxis; (2) telangiectases at characteristic sites; (3) a visceral manifestation; and (4) an affected first-degree relative.

PAVMs may be the first sign of HHT in the presenting patient, and may be the only feature of HHT evident in patients through their thirties, forties, fifties, and beyond. Mucocutaneous telangiectasia are often subtle. Furthermore, the majority of patients

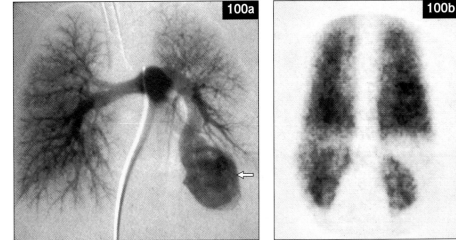

100 Pulmonary arteriovenous malformations. (**a**) Angiographic appearances of pulmonary arteriovenous malformations (arrowed); (**b**) Perfusion scan demonstration of a 40% right-to-left shunt: note the abnormal signal from kidneys, spleen, and liver. Angiogram in (**a**) was performed by Dr James Jackson

will not volunteer a personal or family history of nosebleeds unless specifically asked, and allowed time to check with relatives. Detailed management of the nonpulmonary aspects of HHT is beyond the scope of this text. The importance for the family is that relatives of PAVM patients are likely to have HHT and PAVMs, and be at risk of paradoxical emboli and other complications. Diagnosis of HHT within the family allows presymptomatic screening for PAVMs and treatment before the catastrophic cerebral or haemorrhagic consequences ensue.

HEPATOPULMONARY SYNDROME

Thirty to seventy percent of cirrhotic patients develop intrapulmonary vascular dilatations resulting in right-to-left shunting. The hepatopulmonary syndrome (HPS) was first described as a triad of cirrhosis, clubbing, and cyanosis associated with normal heart and lungs. The syndrome is now defined by the presence of liver disease, an increased $P(A-a)O_2$ breathing room air, and evidence of intrapulmonary vascular dilatations. The anatomical basis appears to be due to dilatation of smaller vessels than usually discussed as representing PAVMs, and embolization therapy is rarely an option. The hypoxaemia and impaired gas transfer recover post-liver transplantation.

Table 68 Causes of haemoptysis

- ❏ **Malignancy**
- ❏ **Inflammation**
  - **TB**
  - **Bronchiectasis including cystic fibrosis**
  - **Suppurative pneumonia**
  - **Aspergilloma**
- ❏ **Pulmonary emboli**
- ❏ **Cardiac causes of pulmonary hypertension**
  - **Acute left ventricular failure**
  - **Mitral stenosis**
- ❏ Vasculitis
- ❏ Anticoagulation
  - Iatrogenic
  - Haematological disorders
- ❏ Trauma
- ❏ Aortic aneurysm
- ❏ Other rare pulmonary causes

Common causes are shown in **bold**

HAEMORRHAGIC CONDITIONS

HAEMOPTYSIS AND MAJOR HAEMORRHAGE

Bleeding can originate from the pulmonary or systemic bronchial circulations. Important causes of haemoptysis are listed in *Table 68*. Pulmonary infarction following pulmonary emboli, and acute inflammatory processes such as suppurative pneumonias, commonly cause less substantial haemoptysis. Major haemorrhage is more likely if abnormal bronchial and pulmonary vascular structures are present.

Abnormal vasculature commonly develops as a result of chronic infective processes. Hypertrophied systemic vessels occur following chronic lung inflammation and infection; conditions such as bronchiectasis and aspergillomas lead to hypertrophied and tortuous bronchial arteries, and transpleural collaterals from intercostal, axillary, and inferior phrenic arteries. Pulmonary artery aneurysms at high risk of rupture, occur particularly in the walls of tuberculous cavities (Rasmussen's aneurysms), lung abscess, and following endovascular seeding from endocarditis and in intravenous drug abusers.

Management of life-threatening haemoptysis

Haemoptysis is life-threatening owing to the possibility of asphyxiation occurring long before systemic hypotension develops. To reduce the risk of asphyxiation, attempts can be made to keep the blood in one lung by nursing the patient on the side suspected of bleeding. Patients should be given high-flow oxygen and fluid, to maintain haemodynamic stability. Expert anaesthetic and ICU support is needed urgently to permit emergency intubation.

Ideally patients should be haemodynamically resuscitated, investigated to assess the site and likely cause of bleeding, then treated. The chest radiograph is extremely helpful in suggesting the side and probable cause – there may not be time for a CT scan. Rigid bronchoscopy under general anaesthesia allows confirmation of the side of bleeding and bronchial suction. However, resuscitation should not delay therapeutic interventions which may be life-saving, even if the bleeding site and diagnosis were not formally established before the procedure was undertaken.

When available, emergency angiography and embolization are usually preferable to emergency thoracic surgery, because of the poor condition of the patient, and the extensive nature of disease when inflamed pleura and transpleural collaterals are present. Unless there are reasons to suspect a pulmonary vascular origin, bronchial angiography and embolization with polyvinyl alcohol particles is usually undertaken first.

Immediate control of bleeding is achieved in the majority of cases, allowing careful discussion of long-term management in a nonemergency situation over the ensuing weeks and months – re-bleeding is likely if the causative pathology is not removed.

ALVEOLAR HAEMORRHAGE AND PULMONARY VASCULITIDES

Alveolar haemorrhage has important consequences for gas exchange whether or not haemoptysis is present. Alveolar haemorrhage is characteristic of pulmonary vascular involvement in the small vessel vasculitides (*Table 69*). Many other rarer primary systemic vasculitides affect the lung vasculature, though pulmonary manifestations are predominantly nonvascular and are discussed in Chapters 7 and 11 (Wegener's disease) and 7 (Churg–Strauss syndrome). Alveolar haemorrhage also occurs in Goodpasture's syndrome, in which the basement membrane is damaged by anti-glomerular basement membrane (anti-GBM) antibodies.

CLINICAL FEATURES

Patients present with dyspnoea, haemoptysis, fever, chest ragiograph changes suggestive of alveolar oedema, and hypoxaemia. The diagnosis is not easy to make, particularly as they are rare (each < 40 cases per million population), and the clinical features of alveolar haemorrhage in an acute inflammatory disorder with elevated CRP and ESR strongly resemble those of pneumonia. Clues to the presence of alveolar haemorrhage and a systemic vasculitic syndrome are obtained from the multi-system involvement, the pattern of disease, the presence of haematuria or urinary activity (casts) on microscopy, and the failure to respond to antibiotics.

The chest radiograph and CT scan both display diffuse alveolar infiltrates, and HR CT scanning using 1 mm slices reveals more disease than is apparent on the chest radiograph. The cardinal sign of alveolar haemorrhage on pulmonary function tests is a supranormal gas transfer factor (DL_{CO} or K_{CO} > 150% predicted) that begins to return to the usual low/normal values soon after commencing treatment. Bronchoscopy can be helpful, as bronchoalveolar lavage should detect haemosiderin-laden macrophages. Diagnostic anti-neutrophil cytoplasmic (ANC) antibodies or anti-GBM antibodies are often present, but lung or renal biopsy may be needed to confirm the diagnosis.

Table 69 Primary vasculitides and alveolar haemorrhage syndromes

	LARGE VESSEL	SMALL VESSEL	OTHER		
	Takayasu's arteritis	Wegener's granulomatosis	Microscopic polyangiitis	Churg–Strauss syndrome	Goodpasture's syndrome
Histological features	Medium/large pulmonary arteries	Necrotizing, granulomatous vasculitis	Capillaritis	Eosinphilic, necrotizing and granulomatous vasculitis	Basement membrane injury
Alveolar haemorrhage	Rare	10%	50%	< 5%	++
Other respiratory symptoms	Usually nil	ENT disease (nasal, sinuses)		Long-standing asthma & rhinitis	Smoking or hydrocarbon triggers
Key non-respiratory disease features	Aorta and branches 'pulseless disease'	Either sex FS glomerulonephritis Systemic features	Either sex Glomerulonephritis (haematuria) Systemic features	Females Eosinophilia Systemic features Cardiac disease	Males Glomerulonephritis
Antibody associations	Usually negative	c-ANCA positive	p-ANCA	p-ANCA	Anti-GBM
Mortality	< 10%	10–20%	10–40%	Low	Low if promptly treated
Treatment	Steroids	Cyclophosphamide and steroids +/– plasmapharesis		Steroids (+/– cyclophos-phamide)	Cyclophosphamide, steroids + plasmapharesis

MANAGEMENT

The mainstay of treatment of these conditions is ventilatory support (oxygenation, noninvasive ventilation, or intubation) and prompt immunosuppression. Steroids are usually sufficient for Churg–Strauss syndrome, but more powerful immunosuppression is needed for Wegener's disease, microscopic polyangiitis, and Goodpasture's syndrome since, in these, untreated or steroid-treated disease leads to death from pulmonary or renal failure within a year in the majority of cases. Goodpasture's syndrome is treated by plasmapharesis to remove the offending antibody, followed by immunosuppression for remission-maintenance. For Wegener's syndrome, cyclophosphamide at 2 mg/kg per day, plus prednisolone 1 mg/kg/day should lead to improvement within a month, though life-threatening pulmonary haemorrhage or renal failure may demand plasmapharesis. Once disease remission is achieved, relapse is common unless prolonged immunosuppression is given. Azathioprine or methotrexate are preferred to cyclophosphamide for remission-maintenance, owing to the severe side-effects of cyclophosphamide (bone marrow suppression and transitional cell carcinomas of the bladder in up 5–10% of treated cases).

CASE STUDIES

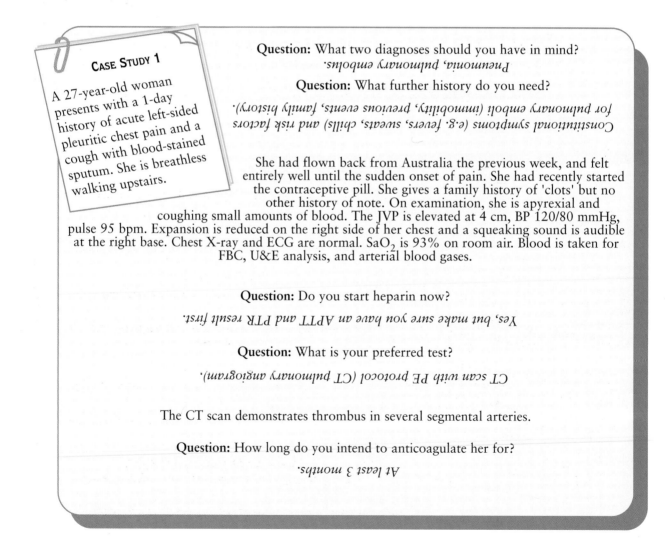

CASE STUDY 1

A 27-year-old woman presents with a 1-day history of acute left-sided pleuritic chest pain and a cough with blood-stained sputum. She is breathless walking upstairs.

Question: What two diagnoses should you have in mind?

Pneumonia, pulmonary embolus.

Question: What further history do you need?

Constitutional symptoms (e.g. fevers, sweats, chills) and risk factors for pulmonary emboli (immobility, previous events, family history).

She had flown back from Australia the previous week, and felt entirely well until the sudden onset of pain. She had recently started the contraceptive pill. She gives a family history of 'clots' but no other history of note. On examination, she is apyrexial and coughing small amounts of blood. The JVP is elevated at 4 cm, BP 120/80 mmHg, pulse 95 bpm. Expansion is reduced on the right side of her chest and a squeaking sound is audible at the right base. Chest X-ray and ECG are normal. SaO$_2$ is 93% on room air. Blood is taken for FBC, U&E analysis, and arterial blood gases.

Question: Do you start heparin now?

Yes, but make sure you have an APTT and PTR result first.

Question: What is your preferred test?

CT scan with PE protocol (CT pulmonary angiogram).

The CT scan demonstrates thrombus in several segmental arteries.

Question: How long do you intend to anticoagulate her for?

At least 3 months.

CASE STUDY 2

You are referred a 40-year-old nonsmoking woman, whose chest radiograph displays a mass in the right lower zone. She was admitted following a minor stroke. She has had nosebleeds since admission, as did her daughter when visiting. On examination, she was cyanosed and clubbed, but otherwise looked well. There were resolving left upper motor neurone signs and no other feature of note except for some red spots on her lips.

Question: What is the differential diagnosis?

PAVM due to hereditary haemorrhagic telangiectasia, complicated by a paradoxical embolic stroke, or lung cancer with cerebral metastases.

A CT scan is requested by your colleague who thinks she has lung cancer. This reveals large vessels entering the lobulated mass.

Question: What would you like to demonstrate on your next test? A perfusion scan demonstrates activity in the kidneys, and the right-to-left shunt is estimated at > 20%.

Confirmation of right-to-left shunting.

Question: In addition to her routine stroke treatments, what two additional treatments does she need?

Antibiotic prophylaxis for dental, surgical, or other invasive procedures. Embolization of pulmonary arteriovenous malformations (performed by an experienced practitioner).

CASE STUDY 3

A 54-year-old nonsmoking man presents with breathlessness. He denies chest pain and was previously fit and well, although he was seeing the ear, nose, and throat surgeon for tests after a 'hole' developed in his nose. On examination, he has a mild pyrexia, the JVP is not elevated, BP is 130/80 mmHg, pulse 98 bpm. He is not cyanosed breathing room air, but the SaO_2 monitor reads 93%. There are bi-basal crackles on examination. The chest radiograph displays fluffy shadowing. The ECG is normal. Your colleague has sent bloods for FBC, U&E, glucose, clotting screen, and cardiac enzymes and is about to give him furosemide.

Question: What diagnosis is your colleague considering?

Pulmonary oedema.

Question: What diagnoses do you think are more likely?

Pulmonary haemorrhage secondary to Wegener's granulomatosis.

Question: What respiratory tests will help you with the diagnosis?

Gas transfer (K_{CO}, DL_{CO}) as part of lung function assessments.

Question: What other tests will help you make the diagnosis?

Urine microscopy for casts, bloods for CRP, ESR, and ANCA, and biopsy of the nose.

SUMMARY

Pulmonary emboli:
- A common disease.
- Missed diagnoses are life-threatening, but PEs are often overdiagnosed.
- They are usually associated with raised JVP and lowered PaO2.
- All patients should have the clinical probability of PE determined before any tests are performed.
- In patients with a low clinical probability of PE, a negative D-dimer test is sufficient to exclude the diagnosis.
- In hypotensive patients, an urgent echocardiogram is the preferred first-line test.
- In normotensive patients, a CT scan is the recommended first-line test.
- A normal CT scan does not exclude the diagnosis of PE.

Pulmonary oedema:
- Is commonly caused by left ventricular failure.
- When cardiac function is normal, consider causes of capillary leak syndrome.
- Diuretics should only be used for hydrostatic pulmonary oedema.

Pulmonary hypertension:
- Clinical features are due to right heart strain and failure.
- Patients usually need oxygen, anticoagulation, and consideration of specific treatments.
- Moderate PH commonly occurs secondary to cardiac or respiratory disease.
- If there is no obvious cause for severe PH, chronic thromboembolic disease must be excluded.
- Primary PH can be treated with vasodilators, but heart–lung transplantation may be needed.

Pulmonary arteriovenous malformations:
- 50% of patients with PAVMs are asymptomatic, but are at risk of stroke and cerebral abscess due to paradoxical emboli.
- Treatment should be considered for all patients to limit complications from PAVMs.
- All patients with PAVMs should receive antibiotic prophylaxis for dental or surgical procedures.
- 80% of PAVM patients will have hereditary haemorrhagic telangiectasia and an 'at risk' family.

Alveolar haemorrhage:
- Is a rare cause of chest radiographic appearances suggestive of pulmonary oedema.
- Can be diagnoses by elevated gas transfer (K_{CO}, DL_{CO}).
- Is usually due to an underlying systemic vasculitis needing immunosuppression.

RECOMMENDED READING

Useful chapters can be found in recent textbooks and British Thoracic Society publications; these provide full lists of primary references. See for example:

Respiratory Medicine, 3rd edn. J. Gibson, D. Geddes, U. Costabel, P. Sterk, B. Corrin (eds). London, Harcourt (2003).

Pulmonary Circulation, 2nd edn. A. Peacock, L. Rubin (eds). London, Arnold (2003).

British Thoracic Society Guidelines for the management of suspected acute pulmonary embolism.British Thoracic Society Standards of Care Committee Pulmonary Embolism Guideline Development Group. *Thorax* 2003;58:470–484.

Chapter 15 Airway pharmacology

INTRODUCTION

This chapter will briefly review theoretical aspects of the classes of commonly used bronchodilators, mediator antagonists, nonsteroid anti-inflammatory drugs (NSAIDs), and corticosteroids. In addition the pharmacology of bronchial challenge will be considered.

CHALLENGE TESTS

BRONCHIAL CHALLENGE

Bronchial challenge is carried out to measure nonspecific bronchial responsiveness, bronchial hyper-responsiveness being a cardinal feature of asthma. It can be used in diagnosis when a patient has normal airway diameter on routine tests (PEF, FEV_1 and so on). It is also used in research. A large number of agents can be used for bronchoprovocation and these are divided into 'direct' acting, which act directly on the bronchial smooth muscle, and 'indirect', which act on intermediate cell(s) subsequently leading to smooth muscle contraction and bronchoconstriction (*Table 70*). Specific bronchial responsiveness refers to specific sensitization to allergens or occupational factors.

As there are a variety of constrictor stimuli available, so the airway response can be measured by a variety of tests of airway calibre. In practice FEV_1 is most commonly used. After initial measurement of FEV_1, saline is administered (to take account of nonspecific responsiveness) and FEV_1 is re-measured and taken as the baseline. Increasing concentrations (usually doubling doses) of the constrictor, e.g. metacholine, are administered, usually by nebulizer, and FEV_1 is re-measured after each. The test is stopped once a 20% fall in FEV_1 has been achieved. The result is expressed (**101**) as the concentration of metacholine, interpolated off the log concentration response curve, necessary to produce a 20% fall in FEV_1 (provocative concentration [PC_{20}] or provocative dose [PD_{20}], calculated from the nebulizer output).

Table 70 Bronchoconstrictor agents which can be used in bronchial challenge

Direct
❑ Pharmacological
   Histamine *
   Metacholine*
   Other cholinergic analogues
   Prostaglandins $PGF_{2\alpha}$, PGD_2
   Leukotrienes LTC_4, LTD_4, LTE_4

Indirect
❑ Pharmacological
   Adenosine monophosphate (AMP)
   Metabisulphite (SO_2)
   Bradykinin
   Neurokinin A
   Propranolol
❑ Physical
   Exercise‡
   Hyperventilation with cold, dry air
   Osmotic: hyper or hypotonic saline
   Distilled water
   Immunological
   – allergens
   – occupational causes

* Most commonly used agents
‡ Commonly used in children

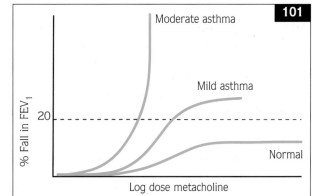

101

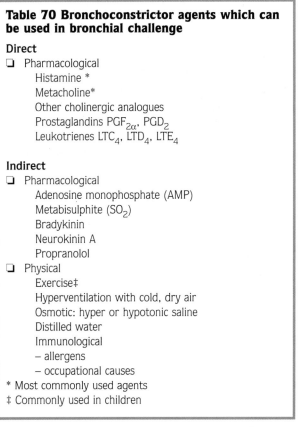

101 Metacholine dose–response curves in bronchial challenge. Reduction in FEV_1 (upwards) occurs with increasing doses of metacholine. A steeper slope is seen in mild asthma compared to a normal subject, such that a 20% fall in FEV_1 occurs in an asthma patient, a level not attained by a normal subject. In both, a plateau effect is seen, when increasing doses of metacholine do not produce further bronchoconstriction. In patients with moderate or severe asthma, the curve is shifted leftwards, i.e. lower doses of metacholine produce greater falls in FEV_1 (lower provocative concentration [PC_{20}]). In addition, the curve no longer plateaus and increased testing may be hazardous to the patient

The shape of the metacholine (or histamine) dose–response curve is altered in asthma: it is shifted to the right, with an earlier take off (lower threshold) and increased slope (bronchial reactivity). The PC_{20} metacholine measures the sensitivity ('twitchiness') of the airways and gives an indication of asthma severity. In addition the response does not plateau with increasing agonist concentrations as it does in normal subjects. There is a loss of limitation of bronchoconstriction in severe asthma. Bronchial responsiveness is increased acutely by factors causing an exacerbation of asthma, by induction of airway inflammation (e.g. by antigen challenge), and it is reduced acutely by an inhaled β_2 agonist and chronically by inhaled steroid therapy, but other drugs, e.g. cromolyns, theophylline, and leukotriene receptor antagonists, have minimal effect.

COUGH CHALLENGE

Cough challenge has been introduced in the laboratory by analogy with bronchial challenge. This remains a research procedure, testing afferent sensitivity of the cough reflex. A variety of agents are used to induce cough, of which capsaicin and citric acid are the most popular.

β_2 ADRENOCEPTOR AGONISTS

Inhaled β_2 agonists are among the most widely used drugs worldwide. Their pharmacology beautifully illustrates general pharmacological principles. They act by binding to β_2 receptors on the cell surface membrane.

β_2 ADRENOCEPTORS

β_2 receptors are a subclass of beta receptors themselves distinguished from alpha adrenoceptors by classical *in vitro* pharmacology (muscle bath experiments using different tissues), structure activity relationships, specific agonists, specific antagonists, and finally genetic analysis and cloning of the actual receptor proteins.

Catecholamines act on α and β receptors, which are divided into subtypes. α receptors are mainly located on arterial smooth muscle and activation of α_1 receptors by sympathetic nervous stimulation, via the neurotransmitter noradrenaline (NA), causes vasoconstriction. α_2 receptors are located presynaptically, and stimulation by NA inhibits sympathetic stimulation, acting as a feedback loop. Very high circulating levels of the hormone adrenaline (usually attained only in hypoglycaemia, post MI or with very heavy exercise) can also activate α_1, α_2, β_1, and β_2 receptors.

β_2 receptors are widely distributed on nearly all cells. The most important are situated on airway smooth muscle, though they are present throughout the lung (*Table 71*). β_1 receptors, however, are of little importance in the lung but are more important in the heart.

Table 71 Lung β_2 and muscarinic receptors: sites and potential pharmacological effects

	Type	Agonist action	Effect	Result
β_2 adrenoceptors				
Airway smooth muscle				
Central	$\beta_1 + \beta_2$	+	Relaxation	Bronchodilatation
Peripheral	β_2		Relaxation	
Vascular smooth muscle	β_2	+	Relaxation	↑VQ mismatch
Endothelium	β_2	+	Inhibition	Antipermeability
Epithelium	β_2	+		Mediators
Mucus glands	β_2	+	Stimulation	
Nerves	β_2	+		
Prejunctional	β_2			
Sensory	β_2	+	Inhibitory	Bronchodilatation
Mast cells	β_2	+	Inhibitory	Reduce mediators
Neutrophils	β_2			
Lymphocytes	β_2			
Cholinergic				
Airway smooth muscle				
(central > peripheral)	M3	+	Inhibitory	Bronchodilatation
Submucosal glands	M3+M1			
Post ganglionic nerves	M2	–	Inhibitory	Limit M3 effects
Airway ganglia	M1	+	Stimulatory	Bronchodilatation

Molecular mechanisms

The β_2 receptor is an archetypal, 7 transmembrane domain structure containing a three-dimensional locus which binds β_2 receptor ligands. β_2 receptor stimulation (**102**) increases intracellular cyclic adenosine monophosphate (cAMP) through a stimulatory coupling G protein (G_s) activating protein kinase A (PKA), which phosphorylates a number of intracellular proteins. PKA directly inhibits myosin light chain kinase and also phosphoinositol hydrolysis, reducing intracellular calcium concentrations. This stimulates a variety of processes leading to smooth muscle relaxation. In addition β_2 agonists, at low concentrations, relax smooth muscle by directly opening membrane potassium channels, mediated via G_s.

The clinical relevance of other potential pulmonary effects due to the stimulation of β_2 receptors on mucus glands, nerves, mast cells, epithelium, endothelium, ciliary function, and inflammatory cells, such as neutrophils and lymphocytes, is unclear but inhibition of mediators and anti-permeability effects could be beneficial (*Table 71*). A broad variety of *in vitro* effects of β_2 stimulation, characterized as 'anti-inflammatory', could be relevant particularly as regards 'nonbronchodilator effects', which are more marked with inhaled long-acting β_2 agonists.

β_2 receptor polymorphisms

A number of β_2 receptor polymorphisms have recently been identified. The two most common variants are characterized by substitution of glycine for arginine at position 16 (Gly-16) and of glutamic acid for glutamine at position 27 (Glu-27) of the extracellular domain of the receptor. *In vitro* homozygous Gly-16 cells are sensitive to β_2 receptor down-regulation whereas homozygous Glu-27 cells are relatively resistant, though β_2 receptor ligand binding is unaltered. *In vivo*, various functional correlates, including asthma severity, nocturnal asthma, bronchial responsiveness, and IgE levels, have been described with different polymorphisms. Two studies have suggested that Arg-16 homozygotes are more susceptible to a reduction in PEF during regular salbutamol treatment. The story is incomplete but offers a potential example of clinically relevant pharmacogenetics.

INHALED β_2 ADRENOCEPTOR AGONISTS

Conventional, inhaled, short-acting β_2 agonists are the most widely used bronchodilators. They produce rapid onset, short-lasting relief of symptoms, particularly breathlessness, and also prevent the development of bronchoconstriction. They are well tolerated.

Dose–response

No other drugs can be administered over such a large dose range without toxicity; 20 µg of salbutamol will produce a bronchodilator effect, although the standard clinical dose is 200 µg, and 10,000 µg (10 mg) is often given by nebulizer. The selectivity conferred by administration by the inhaled route is demonstrated by the fact that 200 µg inhaled is superior to, and less toxic than, a standard oral dose of 4,000 µg.

There are a large number of β_2 agonist drugs which differ in specificity, potency, duration of action, and also the extent to which they are full agonists (producing maximum β_2 receptor effects, e.g. isoprenaline) or partial agonists (such as salbutamol). β receptor blockade is contraindicated in asthma, producing unpredictable, severe, sometimes fatal, bronchoconstriction. Some β receptor blockers, e.g. sotalol, possess partial agonist effects (intrinsic sympathomimetic activity). The importance of these properties in clinical asthma is unclear.

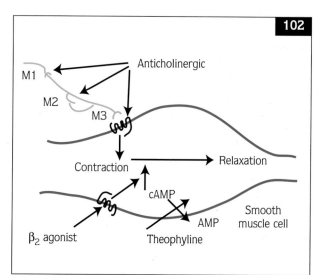

102 Mechanism of action of inhaled β_2 agonists and anticholinergic bronchodilators. AMP, adenosine monophosphate

Side-effects

At conventional doses the usual minor adverse effects of inhaled β_2 agonists include tremor, palpitations, and headaches. These are related to stimulation of β_2 receptors on skeletal muscle, the heart, and vasculature. Tachycardia is produced by activation of β_2 receptors on the peripheral vasculature, producing vasodilatation and a reflex response and stimulation of atrial, chronotropic β_2 receptors, rather than through β_1 receptors, as β_2 agonists are very subtype-specific. At very high doses tachyarrhythmias can occur but these are unusual clinically, as is exacerbation of angina. Hypokalaemia results from β_2 receptor stimulation and intracellular potassium movement. Hyperglycaemia, lactic acidaemia or other metabolic effects are due to effects on liver β_2 and β_3 receptors. Elevation of creatine phosphokinase (CPK) can result from skeletal muscle stimulation.

THE β_2 AGONIST DEBATE

Although considered extremely safe drugs, safety has been a recurring concern because of very wide usage and various 'epidemics' of asthma deaths, often in young people found clutching a reliever inhaler. The first occurrence of an increased death rate was recorded in the 1960s in countries which had recently introduced the first, inhaled, non β_2-selective drugs, isoprenaline and orciprenaline (metaproterenol). Investigation concluded that the deaths were due to severe asthma rather than to cardiac side-effects of β agonist overdose.

However, the recurrence of a marked increase in deaths from asthma, and hospital admissions, particularly in New Zealand, in the 1980s was associated with abuse of the more potent, possibly less selective β_2 agonist, fenoterol. The suggestion was made that fenoterol was prescribed selectively to more severely-affected patients (confounding by severity) but this was refuted by a number of excellent case-control studies and fenoterol was subsequently withdrawn. This remains a contentious matter as there is evidence that asthma severity increased more generally around this time in countries where fenoterol was not widely used, and a reduction in death rates generally accompanied increased prescription of inhaled steroids and improved asthma management.

β_2 AGONIST TOLERANCE

Tachyphylaxis (loss of agonist response due to a reduction in receptor number) is a general phenomenon which has been much studied in the case of β_2 receptors. It occurs owing to rapid receptor phosphorylation, sequestration (internalization and subsequent recirculation), and receptor down-regulation by various mechanisms. This is easily demonstrable *in vitro*. In addition, smooth muscle has been shown to have a very large number of 'spare' β_2 receptors, with a maximal pharmacological response being achieved with activation of only about 5% of the total receptor number.

Tolerance (a higher drug dose being necessary to achieve the same biological effect) is difficult to show *in vivo* because of methodological problems – much lower doses than usually used clinically achieve a near maximal response – and there is confounding from the inherent asthmatic variability and previous β_2 agonist exposure. Careful clinical studies, usually employing a dose–response design, demonstrate a small degree of tolerance to a bronchodilator action of inhaled β_2 agonists but this is of doubtful clinical relevance. More interesting is the more marked effect on loss of bronchoprotection by inhaled β_2 agonists. The beneficial effect of a β_2 agonist inhaled prior to induced bronchoconstriction, whether by exercise or by other bronchial challenge, is lost almost completely after 2 weeks of regular β_2 agonist administration, though the constrictor response is not enhanced.

Clinical studies have now shown that regular four times daily administration of salbutamol is not, *per se*, associated with poor outcome but prescription of a 'reliever' should be as required in contrast to regular treatment with a 'preventer', usually an inhaled steroid. Frequent use of β_2 agonists represents a marker of severe asthma and risk of dying from asthma.

LONG-ACTING INHALED β_2 AGONISTS

Long-acting inhaled β_2 agonists have been the subject of much safety scrutiny. Good clinical studies have confirmed that, co-prescribed with inhaled steroids, salmeterol and formoterol produce better outcomes compared to short-acting β_2 agonists, including improved asthma control and reduced exacerbations of asthma.

Salmeterol is a partial agonist with a high affinity for the β_2 receptor, making it a highly selective β_2 agonist. It has a long backbone of repeating -CH2- groups, making it a highly lipophilic molecule. This allows it to insert itself in the phospholipid bilayer of the cell membrane, resulting in a very long duration of action and perhaps its slow onset of effect. Its ability to re-exert its relaxant effect after being washed off, or displaced from, β_2 receptors on smooth muscle preparations is compatible with the existence of a binding site ('exosite') separate from its active site. It is prescribed at 50–100 µg twice daily.

Formoterol has distinct pharmacological properties (*Table 72*). It is a full agonist with a rapid onset of action (at about 2–3 minutes equivalent to that of salbutamol, compared with 20 minutes for salmeterol). Administration orally does not result in a long duration, suggesting that when inhaled it somehow forms an airway depot, though it is less lipophilic than salmeterol. It has a more obvious dose–response (over 6–24 µg) compared to salmeterol and is given twice daily, but can also be used as a 'reliever'.

ORAL β₂ AGONISTS

Oral β₂ agonists, including slow-release preparations, exist for salbutamol, terbutaline and a pro-drug, bambuterol, which is converted to terbutaline by esterases within the lung. They are used infrequently in the UK because of an adverse risk/benefit ratio with increased side-effects, e.g. tremor, palpitations, and the potential for hypokalaemia and arrhythmias, and reduced benefit compared to administration of lower doses by inhaler. Most patients can find a suitable inhaler device that they can use.

ANTICHOLINERGIC AGENTS

Inhaled anticholinergic bronchodilators are less effective than β₂ agonists in asthma but the reverse may be true in patients with COPD. Anticholinergics act by blocking muscarinic receptors within the airways.

MUSCARINIC RECEPTORS

Parasympathetic cholinergic nerves form the dominant bronchoconstrictor pathway in humans. Post-ganglionic fibres innervate airway smooth muscle, bronchial vessels, and submucosal glands, mainly in the large airways. Sensory afferents in airway epithelium, larynx, and nasopharynx produce reflex bronchoconstriction, maintaining vagal bronchomotor tone. Five different muscarinic receptor subtypes have been cloned and functionally identified in humans but only three exist in the lung. M_1 and M_3 receptors are excitatory and augment ganglionic nicotinic receptors. M_2 receptors are located pre-junctionally at parasympathetic ganglia and on nerve terminals; their activation inhibits acetylcholine release.

The neurotransmitter, acetylcholine, binds to muscarinic M_3 receptors, activating the rapid hydrolysis of phosphoinositol and the formation of inositol 1,4,5 triphosphate. This leads to the release of calcium ions from intracellular stores and contraction of smooth muscle. Inhibition of adenyl cyclase (mediated via M_2 receptors) reduces cAMP concentrations in airway smooth muscle, potentially reducing the effect of β₂ agonist stimulation (**102**). Anticholinergic agents act as competitive antagonists: the effect depends on the dose until maximum blockade is achieved. Older drugs (atropine, ipratropium, and oxitropium) are non-selective, whereas tiotropium, the recently developed once daily, long-acting anticholinergic, is a selective M_1, M_3 receptor antagonist. This is achieved kinetically, as tiotropium dissociates more quickly from M_2 than from M_1 and M_3 receptors.

Table 72 Comparison of inhaled long-acting β₂ agonists

	Salmeterol	Formoterol
β₂ selectivity	++	++
Duration of action	intrinsically long acting	long acting
Agonist activity	partial	full
Onset of action	slow (20 minutes)	rapid (2–3 minutes)
Lipophilicity	++	+
Exosite	+	–
Dose-response	limited	more marked
Indication	preventer	preventer & reliever
Trade name	Serevent	Oxis
Dosage	50–100 µg twice daily	6–24 µg twice daily & 6 µg prn
Inhaler device	MDI, Diskhaler, Accuhaler	Turbohaler
Combination/inhaled steroid	with fluticasone	with budesonide
	Seretide	Symbicort

Side-effects

Older anticholinergic drugs suffer from a bitter taste which, together with their slow onset of action, makes them unpopular with patients. Tiotropium is taken once daily and has no bitter taste. Serious adverse effects are rare but at higher doses pharmacological problems may occur – dry mouth, problems with accommodation, exacerbation of glaucoma or urinary difficulties, particularly in pre-existing prostatic hypertrophy.

THEOPHYLLINES

Theophylline is the most active of the methylxanthines and has been in use as an oral bronchodilator for over 50 years. However, benefits are modest as, despite a variety of slow-release preparations, it may be difficult to achieve adequate, therapeutic plasma concentrations in individual patients. Aminophylline is converted *in vivo* to theophylline, which is the active drug.

The probable mechanism of action is that of phosphodiesterase (PDE) inhibition increasing intracellular cAMP concentrations by inhibiting breakdown. There is no evidence to suggest preferential concentration of these drugs in smooth muscle, and relaxation of smooth muscle is poor at measured plasma therapeutic concentrations. However, other mechanisms may be involved. Both aminophylline and theophylline are nonselective PDE inhibitors. In addition to effects on smooth muscle, anti-inflammatory or immunomodulatory inhibitory effects have been described on eosinophil, lymphocyte, mast cell, and neutrophil function. An increasing number of PDE isoenzymes has been identified; the PDE-4 and PDE-3 subtypes, present in inflammatory cells as well as bronchial smooth muscle, are thought to be the most important. New more specific PDE-3 and PDE-4 inhibitors are at an advanced state of development. Adenosine receptor inhibition may also produce beneficial effects.

Pharmacokinetics

Theophylline is rapidly and totally absorbed from the gastrointestinal tract. Clearance varies considerably between patients, so individual dosing regimens are required with close monitoring of plasma concentration. A therapeutic range of 10–20 mg/l is recommended to achieve bronchodilatation with minimum risk of side-effects, but plasma concentrations below 10 mg/l are associated with clinical response.

Metabolism occurs in the liver predominantly by the cytochrome P450/P448 microsomal enzyme system, which is influenced by a large number of factors.

Metabolism is increased by cigarette smoking and co-administration of enzyme inducers, e.g. anticonvulsants such as phenytoin and carbamazepine. Other drugs reduce metabolism, including antibiotics (e.g. erythromycin, some quinolones) and cimetidine, by inhibiting cytochrome P450. Other factors that reduce hepatic metabolism include ageing, liver disease, heart failure, pneumonia, and certain vaccinations.

Side-effects

Theophylline has a narrow toxic/therapeutic ratio, especially in elderly patients. Side-effects are common, especially with long-term use. Most adverse effects arise through increased dosing but inadequate monitoring of plasma levels and reduced metabolism through co-administration of other drugs may contribute. Common side-effects include gastro-intestinal symptoms, nausea, vomiting, bloating, diarrhoea, headaches, insomnia, arrhythmias, hypokalaemia and, in overdose, convulsions, which may be fatal. Theophylline is poorly tolerated in some individuals even at low doses (and low plasma levels).

CROMOLYNS

Disodium cromoglycate (DSCG) and nedocromil sodium are two inhaled, nonsteroid anti-inflammatory drugs which are now little used in the treatment of asthma. Initially thought to work by inhibiting mast cell mediator release (which they do at high concentration *in vitro*) their mechanism of action is unclear. Inhibition of chloride channels on smooth muscle and/or nerves or inflammatory cells is a possible mode of action.

Clinically they are weak drugs which inhibit a variety of laboratory challenges, including allergen (early and late phase reactions), exercise, meta-bisulphite, AMP, and other indirect-acting stimuli. In asthma therapy they are superior to placebo but equivalent to very low-dose inhaled steroid therapy and have largely been removed from asthma guidelines. DSCG should be taken four times daily though nedocromil is taken twice daily. They have few adverse effects, though DSCG may cause cough.

LEUKOTRIENE RECEPTOR ANTAGONISTS (LTRAS)

Leukotrienes (LTs) are inflammatory mediators with a variety of effects which probably contribute to asthma pathophysiology. The cysteinyl leukotrienes LTC_4 and LTD_4 are the most potent broncho-constrictor agents. LTB_4 is a potent chemotactic agent for inflammatory cells. LTs have been shown to be produced in increased amounts in asthmatic airways. There is particularly strong evidence for their involvement in aspirin-induced asthma (see Chapter 7, page 71).

Arachidonic acid is a ubiquitous component of cell membranes but also the basis of formation of three important classes of mediators – the prostaglandins, thromboxanes, and leukotrienes. Aspirin and other nonsteroidal anti-inflammatory drugs block prostaglandin synthase (cyclo-oxygenase 1 and 2). A number of drugs have been developed to interfere with these biochemical pathways (103). Zileuton is a 5 lipoxygenase inhibitor used in asthma treatment in the US. Two cys-LT receptors – cys-LT$_1$ and cys-LT$_2$ – mediate their actions and a third less well characterized receptor (BLT) mediates LTB$_4$ induced chemotaxis.

Two cys-LT$_1$ receptor antagonists, montelukast and zafirlukast, are currently available in this country (*Table 73*). They are weak bronchodilators but reduce asthma symptoms and β_2 agonist use and also asthma exacerbations. They also reduce circulating eosinophil count. They are equivalent to low-dose inhaled steroid therapy but cannot replace higher doses.

Side-effects

LTRAs are well tolerated with few side-effects and minor drug interactions related to hepatic cytochrome enzyme induction and inhibition. They are used much more in the US, Japan, and some parts of Europe than in the UK. An association with Churg–Strauss syndrome (CSS) has been described with patients, in the vast majority of cases, presenting after the reduction of oral steroid therapy, suggesting that introduction of LTRAs uncovered pre-existing CSS.

CORTICOSTEROIDS

Oral corticosteroids once daily are very effective in the treatment of asthma but cannot be used in the long term because of major toxicity. Prednisolone is the most common oral steroid in use in the UK (prednisone is converted into prednisolone *in vivo*). Synthetic, topically active inhaled corticosteroids were developed to circumvent systemic side-effects. Inhaled steroids currently in use in the UK include:

❏ Beclometasone (BDP).
❏ Budesonide.
❏ Fluticasone.
❏ Mometasone.
❏ Ciclesonide.

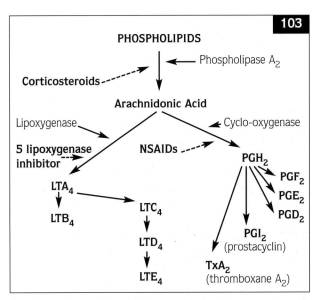

103 Arachidonic acid metabolism and leukotriene modifiers. LT, leukotriene; NSAID, nonsteroidal anti-inflammatory drug; PG, prostaglandin; →, enzymes; −→, inhibitors

Table 73 Comparison of leukotriene receptor antagonist drugs

	Montelukast (MTL)	Zafirlukast
Trade name	Singulair	Accolate
Dosage	10 mg on	20 mg bd
Indication	'Add in' mild–moderate asthma exercise-induced asthma	Treatment of asthma
Age range	Adults Children > 6 y	Adults Children > 12 y
Interactions	CYP 3A4 inducers e.g. rifampicin, phenytoin decrease MTL levels	CYP 2C9 inhibitor warfarin, phenytoin, carbamazepine metabolism

There is conflicting literature (produced mainly by rival pharmaceutical companies) regarding the potency of the different drugs and the efficacy of the different delivery devices employed but there is little to choose as regards efficacy and effectiveness. There is conflicting literature suggesting that the others may potentially be safer than beclometasone (based on a variety of surrogates rather than long-term clinical studies).

Mechanism of action

Glucocorticoid receptors (GR) are present in the cytoplasm of many cell types, and corticosteroids bind to the C terminal end, the N terminal end being concerned with gene transcription. The DNA-binding element consists of two zinc finger projections lying between these two domains. Inactive GR is complexed with two 90 kDa heat shock proteins (hsp90) and other 'chaperone' molecules in the cytoplasm. Corticosteroid binding activates GR with loss of these molecules, allowing translocation into the nucleus and DNA binding as a GR dimer.

Glucocorticoid effects are produced by direct or indirect regulation of transcription of target genes (**104**). GR dimers bind to glucocorticoid response elements (GREs) of DNA on steroid responsive genes, leading to increased or decreased gene repression. GR binds to CREB binding protein at the transcription site, switching on RNA polymerase and increasing protein synthesis e.g. of β_2 receptors. Most of the anti-inflammatory effects of GR result from interaction with transcription factors such as activator protein-1 (AP-1) or nuclear factor-kappa B (NF-kappa B) rather than through negative GREs. Examples of inflammatory genes which are down-regulated by GR in this way include many cytokines, e.g. IL-1, IL-2, IL-3, IL-4, IL-5, IL-6, IL-11, IL-12, IL-13, tumour necrosis factor (TNF) alpha, GMCSF, SCF, chemokines including IL-8, RANTES, eotaxin, MIP-1 alpha, monocyte chemotactic protein-1 (MCP-1), MCP-3, MCP-4, enzymes such as inducible nitric oxide synthase, cyclo-oxygenase 2, and cytoplasmic phospholipase 2, neurokinin receptors, endothelin,

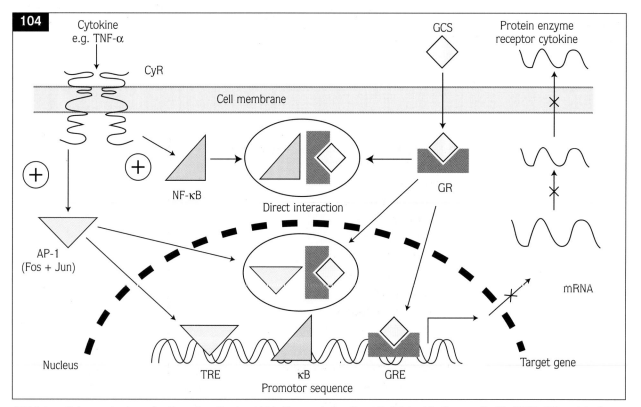

104 Intracellular mechanism of action of corticosteroids (with permission from Dr I Adcock). Glucocorticoids (GCS) diffuse into the cell. AP-1, activator protein 1; CyR, cytoplasmic receptor; GR, glucocorticoid receptor; GRE, glucocorticoid receptor element; mRNA, messenger ribonucleic acid; NF-κB, nuclear factor kappa B; TNF-α, tumour necrosis factor alpha; TRE, transcription response element

and adhesion molecules. This huge array accounts for the enormous spectrum of anti-inflammatory effects involving eosinophils, lymphocytes, mast cells, macrophages, dendritic cells, neutrophils, and epithelial and endothelial cells, all of which seem to be beneficial in treating asthma.

Clinical effects of inhaled steroids

Inhaled corticosteroids are effective in controlling airway inflammation in mild to moderate asthma. There is some evidence that they can decrease but not normalize basement membrane thickening. Inhaled steroids slowly reduce airway hyper-responsiveness (to a variety of stimuli, particularly AMP) but again do not usually result in normalization. In parallel with these effects inhaled steroids have a number of beneficial effects on asthma control (*Table 74*). Unfortunately once inhaled steroids are stopped, most abnormalities reassert themselves rapidly.

Dose-response

In many patients clinical benefit from inhaled steroids appears to plateau at a daily dose of 400 μg BDP equivalent. However, this is a simplistic view, since it will vary not only from patient to patient but in the same patient at different times. Furthermore, the shape of the dose–response will depend on which response is measured and how it is determined. Hence the response of exhaled nitric oxide (NO) will differ from that of symptoms, reliever use, lung function, rate of exacerbations, bronchial responsiveness, and suppression of all the facets of airway inflammation. There is no reason why different parameters should share the same dose–response.

It is well established that higher doses of inhaled steroids are necessary to reduce exacerbations or replace oral steroids than to suppress exhaled NO or improve FEV_1 or PEF. Adding an inhaled long-acting β_2 agonist is more effective than increasing the dose of inhaled steroids as regards asthma control in the majority of patients, but it is not known whether this holds true for reducing airway inflammation. In some patients even large doses of prednisolone fail to improve lung function (see Chapter 7, page 76, Corticosteroid resistance).

Side-effects

Adverse effects are common with continuous prednisolone but uncommon at low doses of inhaled steroids and are more feared than real (see Chapter 7, page 63).

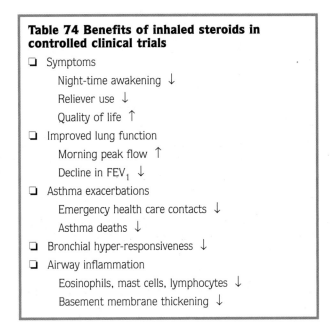

Table 74 Benefits of inhaled steroids in controlled clinical trials

❑ Symptoms
     Night-time awakening ↓
     Reliever use ↓
     Quality of life ↑
❑ Improved lung function
     Morning peak flow ↑
     Decline in FEV_1 ↓
❑ Asthma exacerbations
     Emergency health care contacts ↓
     Asthma deaths ↓
❑ Bronchial hyper-responsiveness ↓
❑ Airway inflammation
     Eosinophils, mast cells, lymphocytes ↓
     Basement membrane thickening ↓

Note: answers are on page 176

1 IN A SMOKER WITH COPD WHICH IS TRUE?
A Oxygen saturation measured with a pulse oximeter may be falsely high.
B Total lung capacity is usually below predicted.
C A single peak flow reading clinches the diagnosis.
D After bronchodilators an improvement of about 30% in FEV_1 is expected.

2 WHAT ARE THE FEATURES OF RIGHT UPPER LOBE COLLAPSE?
A Pleural effusion.
B Elevation of right hilar structures.
C Elevation of right hemidiaphragm.
D The 'sail' sign.
E Mediastinal shift to the left.

3 WHICH OF THE FOLLOWING STATEMENTS IS TRUE?
A Lung cancer is the commonest cancer in women.
B Lung cancer is the commonest cause of cancer death in women.
C 50% of lung cancers are caused by smoking.
D Stopping smoking can reduce the risk of lung cancer in 2 years.
E Asbestos exposure is the only occupational carcinogen that increases lung cancer risk.

4 WHICH OF THE FOLLOWING STATEMENTS IS TRUE?
A Small-cell lung cancer is more common than nonsmall-cell cancer.
B Squamous cell types are much more common than adenocarcinoma.
C Adenocarcinoma is the cell type most associated with smoking.
D Squamous cell carcinoma has the slowest cell doubling time.
E Large-cell carcinoma has the fastest cell doubling time.

5 WHICH OF THE FOLLOWING STATEMENTS IS TRUE?
A Surgery is the treatment of choice for small cell cancer.
B Surgery is the treatment of choice for NSCLC stage II or less.
C Surgery is the treatment of choice for NSCLC stage III.
D Surgery is the treatment of choice for NSCLC stage IV.
E All patients should have a CT brain scan before curative surgery.

6 THE FOLLOWING ARE KNOWN TO IMPROVE MORTALITY IN COPD:
A Inhaled bronchodilators.
B Nebulized bronchodilators.
C Long-term oxygen therapy.
D Oral steroids.
E Pulmonary rehabilitation.

7 USUAL TREATMENTS FOR AN ACUTE EXACERBATION OF COPD ARE:
A 100% oxygen.
B Antiviral agents.
C Inhaled steroids.
D Oral steroids.
E Antibiotics.

8 SMOKING CESSATION:
A After the age of 55 has no effect on COPD.
B Is more effective than bronchodilators as a long-term treatment for COPD.
C Is better achieved with nicotine patches than chewing gum.
D Is better achieved by a combination of bupropion and NRT than either alone.
E Is never achieved simply by just giving advice, however personalized.

9 LONG-TERM OXYGEN THERAPY IN COPD:
A Is best provided via an oxygen concentrator.
B Is usually provided as part of a pulmonary rehabilitation programme.
C Is of proven benefit in smokers and nonsmokers.
D Is of value even if used for 8 hours a day.
E Is best started during a stay in hospital with an acute exacerbation.

10 IN ACUTE SEVERE ASTHMA WHICH OF THESE STATEMENTS IS TRUE?
A The onset is usually sudden.
B The $PaCO_2$ is usually elevated.
C Intravenous hydrocortisone is always indicated.
D Nebulized ipratropium is the bronchodilator of choice.
E Intravenous magnesium may be indicated.

11 IN THE DAY-TO-DAY MANAGEMENT OF ADULT ASTHMA WHICH OF THESE STATEMENTS IS TRUE?

A   Regular need for an inhaled bronchodilator more than once daily indicates prescription of a preventer therapy (usually an inhaled steroid).

B   A trial of a high-dose inhaled steroid (BDP equivalent > 2,000 µg daily) should always be undertaken before prescribing a long-acting inhaled β_2 agonist.

C   Leukotriene receptor antagonists are the mainstay of treatment.

D   Theophylline may be useful but should be reserved for use at steps 4 and 5.

12 THE FOLLOWING MEDICATIONS MAY MAKE ASTHMA WORSE:

A   Aspirin.

B   Amoxicillin.

C   Aminophylline.

D   Timolol eye drops.

13 WHICH OF THE FOLLOWING STATEMENTS IS TRUE OF SARCOIDOSIS?

A   Is milder in Afro-Caribbeans than in Caucasians.

B   Is caused by infection with a hitherto unidentified micro-organism.

C   Is characterized histologically by accumulation of B lymphocytes in affected organs.

D   Affects the lungs in 60% of cases.

E   Does not require treatment when the patient has no symptoms or lung function abnormalities.

14 WHICH OF THE FOLLOWING STATEMENTS IS TRUE IN CRYPTOGENIC FIBROSING ALVEOLITIS?

A   Is commoner in women than in men.

B   Correlates pathologically with usual interstitial pneumonitis.

C   Is characterized by insidious onset of cough and breathlessness.

D   Typically causes a restrictive ventilatory defect.

E   Commonly progresses to type II respiratory failure.

15 WHICH OF THE FOLLOWING STATEMENTS IS TRUE OF ASBESTOSIS?

A   Is the only respiratory disease caused by exposure to asbestos.

B   Is one of at least four different respiratory diseases caused by inhaled asbestos.

C   Typically develops 15–20 years after exposure to asbestos.

D   Is generally rapidly progressive.

E   Responds well to oral corticosteroids.

16 WHICH OF THE FOLLOWING STATEMENTS IS TRUE OF EXTRINSIC ALLERGIC ALVEOLITIS?

A   Can be acute, subacute, or chronic.

B   Can result from exposure to mouldy hay.

C   Does not result from exposure to parakeets.

D   Is associated with the presence of circulating IgG antibodies.

E   Never requires steroid treatment if antigen exposure can be avoided.

17 THE FOLLOWING SUGGEST AN EXUDATE:

A   Pleural fluid protein > 30 g/l.

B   Pleural fluid protein < 30 g/l.

C   Pleural fluid LDH > 200 IU.

D   Pleural fluid protein:serum protein ratio > 0.5.

E   Pleural fluid protein:serum protein ratio < 0.5.

18 EMPYEMA:

A   Can be a medical emergency.

B   Is indicated by serous pleural fluid.

C   Microbiological confirmation should be sought as soon as possible.

D   Pleural fluid LDH is < 200 IU.

E   Surgery is rarely indicated.

19 WHICH OF THE FOLLOWING STATEMENTS IS TRUE OF PNEUMOTHORAX?

A   Spontaneous pneumothoraces are more common in women.

B   Spontaneous pneumothoraces are more common in tall people.

C   Spontaneous pneumothoraces are rarely seen in people under 40 years old.

D   All pneumothoraces require intercostal tube drainage.

E   To confirm the presence of a tension pneumothorax an urgent chest X-ray is essential.

20 IN INFECTIONS OF THE UPPER RESPIRATORY TRACT:

A   Epiglottitis is associated with a risk of fatal upper airway obstruction.

B   Amoxicillin is the empirical treatment of choice.

C   Zanamivir prevents influenza in susceptible adults.

D   Nebulized budesonide may be of value.

E   Vaccination against the flu is recommended in post splenectomy patients.

21 COMMUNITY-ACQUIRED PNEUMONIA IS:

A   Best treated in hospital.

B   Likely to have a poorer outcome in patients with a diastolic blood pressure < 70 mmHg.

C   Most commonly caused by pneumococcus (*Streptococcus pneumoniae*).

D   Best treated after accurate identification of the organism causing the infection.

E   Associated with a higher mortality in patients requiring admission to the intensive care unit.

22 IN AN IMMUNOCOMPROMISED HOST:

A *Pneumocystis jiroveci* is the commonest cause of pneumonia.

B Ganciclovir can be used as prophylaxis against cytomegalovirus infection.

C Pneumonia is always accompanied by some respiratory symptoms or signs.

D A bronchoalveolar lavage (BAL) is a useful tool in the diagnosis of pneumonia.

E *Aspergillus* infections are particularly common in HIV patients.

23 WHICH OF THE FOLLOWING STATEMENTS IS TRUE OF TUBERCULOSIS?

A Is diagnosed by a Mantoux test.

B Requires treatment for 3 months for a complete cure.

C Of the genitourinary tract is the commonest form of nonpulmonary TB.

D Is commoner in patients with cystic fibrosis.

E In immigrants is usually due to infection acquired in the UK.

24 THE FOLLOWING ARE CAUSES OF BRONCHIECTASIS:

A Cystic fibrosis.

B Muscular dystrophy.

C Pertussis infection.

D α-1 antitrypsin deficiency.

25 PATIENTS WITH CYSTIC FIBROSIS:

A Are usually diagnosed in childhood.

B Rarely live beyond 20 years of age.

C Have an increased risk of diabetes.

D Have a sweat chloride concentration of < 20 mmol/l.

26 OBSTRUCTIVE SLEEP APNOEA:

A Is more common in women.

B May cause poor quality sleep.

C Is a cause of car crashes.

D Nasal continuous positive airway pressure is an effective treatment.

27 RESPIRATORY FAILURE CAN BE ASSOCIATED WITH:

A High arterial carbon dioxide levels.

B A high respiratory rate (> 20 breaths/min).

C Cyanosis.

D An elevated alveolar–arterial oxygen gradient.

E Loss of consciousness.

28 THE FOLLOWING CHARACTERISTICALLY CAUSE TYPE II RESPIRATORY FAILURE:

A Pneumonia.

B Exacerbations of COPD.

C Motor neurone disease.

D Pulmonary embolism.

E Acute severe asthma.

29 NONINVASIVE VENTILATION IS:

A Contra-indicated in unconscious patients.

B Delivered through an endotracheal tube.

C Useful in the management of acute exacerbations of COPD.

D Not compatible with supplemental oxygen therapy.

E Helpful in patients with respiratory failure due to pulmonary embolism.

30 INHALED β$_2$ AGONISTS:

A Show little dose-response.

B Produce tremor.

C Are more effective than anticholinergics in asthma.

D Demonstrate tolerance.

31 THEOPHYLLINE:

A Has a wide therapeutic/toxic ratio.

B Is useful by rectal administration.

C Is expensive.

D Is as effective as doubling the dose of inhaled steroids.

32 STEROIDS:

A Increase gene transcription.

B Act to inhibit genes via transcription factors.

C By inhalation increase bronchial responsiveness.

D By inhalation can reduce blood eosinophil counts.

33 A 24-YEAR-OLD PATIENT IS CYANOSED AND CLUBBED. POSSIBLE DIAGNOSES INCLUDE:

A Hepatopulmonary syndrome.

B Pulmonary arteriovenous malformation.

C Eisenmenger's syndrome.

D Cyanotic congenital heart disease that has been treated by surgery.

E Pulmonary emboli.

Index

Page numbers in **bold** refer to major coverage of a topic; those in *italic* refer to tables

True answers

1	A	**12**	A, D	**23**	None
2	B, C	**13**	E	**24**	A, C, D
3	B	**14**	B, C, D	**25**	A, C
4	D	**15**	B, C	**26**	B, C, D
5	B	**16**	A, B, D	**27**	All of these
6	C	**17**	A, C, D	**28**	B, C
7	D, E	**18**	A, C, E	**29**	A, C
8	B, D	**19**	B	**30**	B, C, D
9	A	**20**	A, D	**31**	D
10	E	**21**	C, E	**32**	A, D
11	A, D	**22**	B, D	**33**	A, B, C, D